# New Diagnostic and Therapeutic Tools in Child Neurology

# Mariani Foundation Paediatric Neurology Series
*Editorial Board*

Giuliano Avanzini, Milan, Italy
Philippe Evrard, Paris, France
Raoul Hennekam, Amsterdam, The Netherlands
Eugenio Mercuri, Rome, Italy
Fabio Sereni, Milan, Italy
Lawrence Wrabetz, Milan, Italy

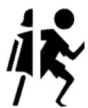

Fondazione Pierfranco e Luisa Mariani
Viale Bianca Maria 28
20129 Milan, Italy

Telephone: +39 02 795458
Fax: +39 02 76009582
e-mail: publications@fondazione-mariani.org
www.fondazione-mariani.org

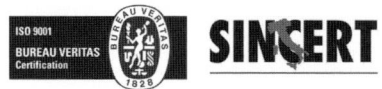

# New Diagnostic and Therapeutic Tools in Child Neurology

*Edited by*

Eugenio Mercuri,
Ermellina Fedrizzi and Giovanni Cioni

**Mariani Foundation Paediatric Neurology Series: 24**
**Series founder: Maria Majno**
Associate editor: Valeria Basilico

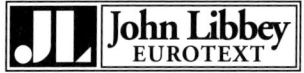

ISSN: 0969-0301
ISBN: 978-2-7420-0813-1

*Cover illustration*: *Figure and Birds*, Joan Miró, 1948. © Successió Miró/ADAGP, Paris, by SIAE, 2011.

*Technical and language editor:* Justine Cullinan.

Published by

**Éditions John Libbey Eurotext**
127, avenue de la République, 92120 Montrouge, France
Tél. : +33 (0)1 46 73 06 60
Fax : +33 (0)1 40 84 09 99
e-mail : contact@jle.com
www.jle.com

© 2011 John Libbey Eurotext. All rights reserved.

Unauthorized duplication contravenes applicable laws.

It is prohibited to reproduce this work or any part of it without authorization of the publisher or of the Centre Français d'Exploitation du Droit de Copie (CFC), 20, rue des Grands-Augustins, 75006 Paris, France.

# Contents

| | | |
|---|---|---:|
| Chapter 1 | Effect of treatment of subclinical neonatal seizures detected with amplitude-integrated electroencephalography: randomized, controlled trial<br>*Linda G.M. van Rooij, Mona C. Toet, Alexander C. van Huffelen, Floris Groenendaal, Wijnand Laan, Alexandra Zecic, Timo de Haan, Irma L.M. van Straaten, Sabine Vrancken, Gerda van Wezel, Jaqueline van der Sluijs, Henk ter Horst, Danilo Gavilanes, Sabrina Laroche, Gunnar Naulaers and Linda S. de Vries* | 1 |
| Chapter 2 | Neurologic assessment and cerebral MRI in preterm infants<br>*Licia Lugli, Isotta Guidotti, Natascia Bertoncelli and Fabrizio Ferrari* | 15 |
| Chapter 3 | Neuroimaging techniques: general concepts<br>*Luca A. Ramenghi* | 25 |
| Chapter 4 | Diffusion MR techniques to study the neonatal brain<br>*Nora Tusor, Serena Counsell and Mary Rutherford* | 33 |
| Chapter 5 | Visual development: new tools for assessment in the neonatal period<br>*Daniela Ricci, Domenico Romeo and Eugenio Mercuri* | 55 |
| Chapter 6 | Brain transcranial stimulation: diagnostic and therapeutic applications<br>*Federico Ranieri, Paolo Profice, Fabio Pilato, Fioravante Capone, Lucia Florio, Michele Dileone and Vincenzo Di Lazzaro* | 63 |
| Chapter 7 | High-density electroencephalography<br>*Giuliano Avanzini and Ferruccio Panzica* | 73 |
| Chapter 8 | Diagnosis of auditory processing disorders<br>*Elisabetta Genovese, Mariavittoria Vallarino, Maria Consolazione Guarnaccia and Daniele Monzani* | 83 |
| Chapter 9 | Muscle MRI: phenotype–genotype correlation<br>*Eugenio Mercuri, Flaviana Bianco, Gessica Vasco and Marika Pane* | 91 |

Chapter 10   Functional MRI in children: clinical applications
             *Andrea Zsoter and Martin Staudt*                                          97

Chapter 11   Clinical and instrumental assessment of the upper limb in cerebral palsy
             *Giuseppina Sgandurra and Giovanni Cioni*                                 107

Chapter 12   Robotics and rehabilitation: new perspectives
             *Stefano Mazzoleni, Paolo Dario and Maria Chiara Carrozza*                121

# Chapter 1

# Effect of treatment of subclinical neonatal seizures detected with amplitude-integrated electroencephalography: randomized, controlled trial*

Linda G.M. van Rooij[a], Mona C. Toet[a], Alexander C. van Huffelen[b], Floris Groenendaal[a], Wijnand Laan[c], Alexandra Zecic[d], Timo de Haan[e], Irma L.M. van Straaten[f], Sabine Vrancken[g], Gerda van Wezel[h], Jaqueline van der Sluijs[i], Henk ter Horst[j], Danilo Gavilanes[k], Sabrina Laroche[l], Gunnar Naulaers[m] and Linda S. de Vries[a]

Departments of [a]Neonatology and [b]Clinical Neurophysiology, Wilhelmina Children's Hospital, and [c]Julius Centre for Health Sciences and Primary Care, University Medical Centre Utrecht, Utrecht, Netherlands;
[d]Department of Neonatology, University Hospital Ghent, Ghent, Belgium;
[e]Department of Neonatology, Academic Medical Centre Amsterdam, Amsterdam, Netherlands;
[f]Department of Neonatology, Isala Clinics Zwolle, Zwolle, Netherlands;
[g]Department of Neonatology, University Medical Centre St Radboud Nijmegen, Nijmegen, Netherlands;
[h]Department of Neonatology, Leiden University Medical Centre, Leiden, Netherlands;
[i]Department of Neonatology, Maxima Medical Centre Veldhoven, Veldhoven, Netherlands;
[j]Department of Neonatology, University Medical Centre Groningen, Groningen, Netherlands;
[k]Division of Neonatology, Department of Pediatrics, University Hospital Maastricht, Maastricht, Netherlands;
[l]Department of Neonatology, University Hospital Antwerp, Antwerp, Belgium;
[m]Department of Neonatology, University Hospital Leuven, Leuven, Belgium
l.s.devries@umcutrecht.nl

* This trial has been registered at the International Standard Randomized Controlled Trial Number Registry (identifier ISRCTN61541169) and is reprinted with permission from *Pediatrics*, Vol. 125, pp. 358–366. Copyright © 2010 by the AAP. This article was originally published online Jan 25, 2010 and can be found at <http://www.pediatrics.org/cgi/content/full/125/2/e358>
DOI: 10.1542/peds.2009-0136

## Summary

Seizures are common in full-term infants with hypoxic-ischaemic encephalopathy (HIE). A substantial portion of neonatal seizures are subclinical. There is concern about possible adverse effects of neonatal seizures on the immature brain. The objectives of this study were to investigate how many subclinical seizures in full-term neonates with HIE would be missed without continuous amplitude-integrated electroencephalography (aEEG) and whether immediate treatment of both clinical and subclinical seizures would result in a reduction in the total duration of seizures and a decrease in brain injury, as seen on MRI scans. In this multicentre, randomized, controlled trial, term infants with moderate to severe HIE and subclinical seizures were assigned randomly to either treatment of both clinical seizures and subclinical seizure patterns (group A) or blinding of the aEEG registration and treatment of clinical seizures only (group B). All recordings were reviewed with respect to the duration of seizure patterns and the use of antiepileptic drugs (AEDs). MRI scans were scored for the severity of brain injury. Nineteen infants in group A and 14 infants in group B were available for comparison. Results showed that the median duration of seizure patterns in group A was 196 minutes, compared with 503 minutes in group B (not statistically significant). No significant differences in the number of AEDs were seen. Five infants in group B received AEDs when no seizure discharges were seen on aEEG traces. Six of 19 infants in group A and 7 of 14 infants in group B died during the neonatal period. A significant correlation between the duration of seizure patterns and the severity of brain injury in the blinded group, as well as in the whole group, was found. It was concluded that in this small group of infants with neonatal HIE and seizures, there was a trend for a reduction in seizure duration when clinical and subclinical seizures were treated. The severity of brain injury seen on MRI scans was associated with a longer duration of seizure patterns.

## Introduction

Neonatal seizures are common in full-term infants with hypoxic-ischaemic encephalopathy (HIE) and pose a high risk for death or neurologic disability (McBride *et al.*, 2000; Miller *et al.*, 2002; Scher *et al.*, 1989; Volpe, 2001). Clinical recognition of neonatal seizures may be difficult, because manifestations may be subtle (Volpe, 2001). Conventional electroencephalography (cEEG) is the standard method to confirm neonatal seizures. Unfortunately, this tool has its limitations; in most units, equipment, technicians, and experienced clinical neurophysiologists are not available 24 hours per day. In the past decade, amplitude-integrated electroencephalography (aEEG) has become a bedside tool that is now used routinely in many NICUs. Prolonged monitoring with aEEG as well as continuous video electroencephalography (EEG) has shown that a substantial proportion of neonatal seizures are subclinical, especially after administration of antiepileptic drugs (AEDs) (Boylan *et al.*, 2002; Clancy *et al.*, 1988; Lawrence *et al.*, 2009; Mizrahi & Kellaway, 1987; Scher *et al.*, 2003). Because clinical recognition of neonatal seizures is difficult, the presence of clinical seizures may be overestimated, resulting in unnecessary use of AEDs. Conversely, subclinical neonatal seizures may not be recognized without continuous monitoring, resulting in inadequate treatment (Lawrence *et al.*, 2009; Murray *et al.*, 2008). Although human data are scarce, studies suggest an adverse effect of both clinical and subclinical seizures on neurodevelopmental outcomes. Neonatal seizures have been reported to predispose patients to later problems with regard to cognition, behavior, and development of postneonatal epilepsy (McBride *et al.*, 2000; Miller *et al.*, 2002; Levene, 2002). Although there is potential harm of seizures in the immature brain, there also is concern about possible adverse effects of anticonvulsant medications on the developing brain (Bittigau *et al.*, 2002, 2003; Sicca *et al.*, 2000). Previous studies showed that infants treated for clinical and subclinical seizures had a lower incidence of postneonatal epilepsy, compared with those treated only for clinical seizures (Brunquell *et al.*, 2002; Clancy & Legido, 1991; Hellström-Westas *et al.*, 1995; Toet *et al.*, 2005). This was one of the reasons we performed this randomized, controlled trial to investigate whether immediate treatment of both clinical and subclinical seizures detected with continuous aEEG resulted in reduction of the total duration of seizures and less-severe brain injury seen on MRI scans.

## Methods

### Study design

We conducted a randomized, prospective, multicentre trial (Subclinical Seizure Question [Suseque] Study). Eleven perinatal centres in the Netherlands and Belgium participated between November 2003 and April 2008. All participating centres were trained in the application and interpretation of aEEG and followed a standardized study protocol. The institutional review board of every centre approved the protocol. Written informed consent was obtained from parents before randomization.

### Entry criteria

Infants were eligible for the study on the basis of gestational age of $\geq 37$ weeks, admission to 1 of the NICUs $< 24$ hours after birth, and diagnosis of HIE and neonatal seizures. HIE was defined on the basis of meeting $\geq 3$ of the following criteria: (1) signs of intrauterine asphyxia (*i.e.*, late decelerations on fetal electrocardiograms or meconium-stained liquor), (2) arterial cord blood pH of $< 7.10$, (3) delayed onset of spontaneous respiration, (4) Apgar score of $\leq 5$ at 5 minutes, or (5) multiorgan failure (elevated liver enzyme levels, reduced diuresis, and cardiovascular problems).

Exclusion criteria included the presence of congenital or chromosomal abnormalities, maternal use of narcotics or sedatives, treatment with phenytoin before referral, and administration of muscle-relaxing drugs. Infants who demonstrated subclinical status epilepticus at the beginning of the aEEG registration also were excluded because immediate treatment with AEDs was considered indicated.

### Randomization

For infants who met the entry criteria, aEEG was started immediately after admission. If infants demonstrated clinical seizures, then they were treated with AEDs. When infants showed their first subclinical seizure, as confirmed with aEEG, they were assigned randomly to either group A (treatment of both clinical and subclinical seizure patterns) or group B (blinding of the aEEG registration and treatment of only clinical seizures). We stratified randomization according to centre with a randomized block design with a block size of 6. Randomization codes for every centre were supplied in numbered sealed envelopes.

### aEEG monitoring

aEEG was performed with an Olympic 6000 cerebral function monitor (Natus, Seattle, WA). Single-channel aEEG signals were recorded from 2 parietal needle electrodes (corresponding to P3 and P4 in the International 10–20 System). The EEG signal was filtered, rectified, and smoothed before it was printed out at slow speed (6 cm/hour). A second tracing recorded the electrode impedance continuously. The Olympic 6000 monitor gave access to the raw EEG data in the review mode and, with the latest software version, the raw EEG signal ran continuously during recording. For blinding of the screen, we used special software (Olympic Medical, Seattle, WA). During blinding, the impedance recording was visible and events such as care procedures, medications, and clinical seizures could be marked.

## Treatment protocol

Table 1 shows the treatment protocol. In the first years (November 2003 to June 2005), lidocaine was given as a second-line drug. Because of concerns about potential cardiovascular side effects and the fact that midazolam was sometimes used around the time of intubation, we changed our treatment protocol (Malingré et al., 2006), with midazolam being given as the second AED. Twenty-six infants received midazolam as a second drug.

## Grading of HIE

HIE was classified as moderate (grade II) or severe (grade III) according to the criteria described by Sarnat & Sarnat (1976). Evaluation of HIE took place 24 and 48 hours after birth.

## aEEG analysis

Seizure patterns (characteristic pattern, with a sudden increase of both minimal and maximal amplitudes of the recorded signal and a decrease in amplitude in the postictal period) were classified (Hellström-Westas & Rosen, 2006) as a single seizure pattern, repetitive seizures ($\geqslant$ 3 seizure patterns during a 30-minute period), or status epilepticus (continuous seizure pattern for $\geqslant$ 30 minutes, presenting as a 'sawtooth pattern' or as continuous increases of the lower and upper margins). All aEEG recordings were analyzed off-line after the completion of enrollment. Analysis was performed independently by 2 aEEG experts (Drs de Vries and Toet), with respect to seizure patterns and background pattern. The readers had full access to all marked events, for differentiation between true ictal discharges and artifacts. When there was disagreement about seizure discharges or background patterns between the 2 raters, a third rater (Dr van Rooij) was involved and consensus was reached.

For each infant, the total duration of seizures was calculated (in minutes) by using the raw EEG data. When status epilepticus was seen, this was taken as 1 period. Only seizure patterns that could be confirmed with the raw EEG data were selected. When AEDs were given, we assessed whether treatment was appropriate, meaning that AEDs were given within 2 hours after the onset of clinical and/or subclinical seizures and another AED was administered if no effect was seen within 1 to 2 hours. For infants in group B, who received AEDs for clinical seizures, we analyzed the aEEG findings for the presence of EEG seizure patterns at the time when clinical seizures were observed.

Table 1. Treatment protocol for neonatal seizures

| Step | Treatment |
|---|---|
| 1 | Phenobarbitone: 20 mg/kg, eventually another 10 mg/kg |
| 2[a] | Midazolam: loading dose of 0.05 mg/kg, followed by continuous infusion of 0.15 mg/kg per h, to maximum of 0.2 mg/kg per h (when seizures have been stopped for 24 h, tapered to 0.1 mg/kg per h and stopped after 48 h) |
| 3[a] | Lidocaine: loading dose of 2 mg/kg, followed by continuous infusion of 6 mg/kg per h for 6 h, then 4 mg/kg per h for 12 h, and then 2 mg/kg per h for 12 h (always stopped after 36 h) |
| 4[a] | Clonazepam: loading dose of 0.1 mg/kg, followed by continuous infusion of 0.1–0.5 mg/kg per d |
| 5[a] | Pyridoxine: 50 mg/kg |
| 6[a] | Further treatment on basis of clinician's decision |

[a] Every next step is taken when no effect is seen within 1 to 2 hours after administration of the AED or when recurrence of seizures is noted.

## MRI scoring

Depending on their clinical condition, infants underwent MRI 4 to 10 days after birth. MRI scans were reviewed retrospectively by 2 investigators (Drs Groenendaal and de Vries), who were blinded to aEEG results. The severity of brain injury was assessed by using conventional T1- and T2-weighted spin echo sequences, with diffusion-weighted imaging and apparent diffusion coefficient maps when available. Injury was scored for the basal ganglia and thalami in combination with cortical involvement, the watershed areas, and the posterior limb of the internal capsule, by using systems described previously as being predictive for neurodevelopmental outcomes after HIE22–24 (Barkovitch et al., 1998; Rutherford et al., 1998; Shah et al., 2006) (Table 2).

Table 2. Scoring system for brain injury seen on MRI scans

| Score | Description |
|---|---|
| Basal ganglia and thalamus | |
| 0 | Normal |
| 1 | Abnormal signal in thalamus |
| 2 | Abnormal signal in thalamus and lentiform nucleus |
| 3 | Abnormal signal in thalamus, lentiform nucleus and perirolandic cortex |
| 4 | More-extensive involvement |
| Watershed areas | |
| 0 | Normal |
| 1 | Single focal infarction |
| 2 | Abnormal signal in anterior or posterior watershed white matter |
| 3 | Abnormal signal in anterior or posterior watershed cortex and white matter |
| 4 | Abnormal signal in both anterior and posterior watershed zones |
| 5 | More-extensive cortical involvement |
| Posterior limb of internal capsule | |
| 0 | Myelination present |
| 1 | Myelination present but impaired |
| 2 | Myelination absent |

## Statistical analyses

Before the study was started, a power analysis was performed by using a power $(1 - \beta)$ of .80 and a significance level ($\alpha$) of .05. This resulted in a sample size of 65 infants in both groups.

Statistical analysis was performed by using SPSS 12.0 for Windows (SPSS Inc, Chicago, IL). Comparisons of baseline and aEEG characteristics between groups were made with Fisher's exact test or $\chi^2$ tests for categorical variables and with $t$ tests for logarithmically transformed continuous variables. Univariate linear regression models were used to test differences in the duration of seizure patterns between groups and to evaluate the association between seizure duration and MRI scores. The level of significance was set at .05.

## Results

**Baseline characteristics**

During the study period, a total of 138 infants met the inclusion criteria (Fig. 1). Neonatal baseline characteristics are summarized in Table 3. There were no substantial differences between groups regarding clinical characteristics. One infant also had a right-sided middle cerebral artery infarction and a left-sided anterior cerebral artery infarction. None of the infants received hypothermia as treatment for HIE.

**aEEG characteristics**

aEEG characteristics are summarized in Table 4. These characteristics were not statistically different between treatment arms.

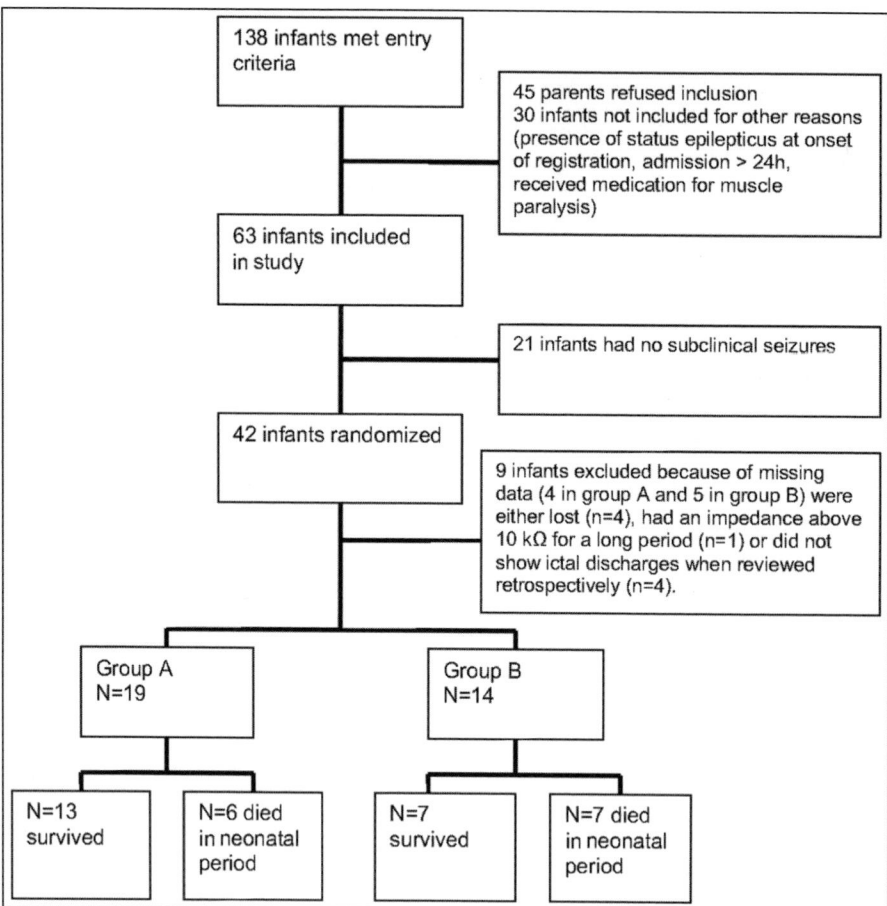

*Fig. 1. Flow diagram of inclusion.*

Table 3. Baseline characteristics

| | Group A (N = 19) | Group B (N = 14) | Total (N = 33) |
|---|---|---|---|
| Gestational age, mean ± SD, wk | 39.5 ± 1.8 | 39.9 ± 1.3 | 39.7 ± 1.6 |
| Birth weight, mean ± SD, g | 3,254 ± 701 | 3,416 ± 487 | 3,320 ± 620 |
| Gender, n (%) | | | |
| Male | 8 (42) | 7 (50) | 15 (46) |
| Female | 11 (58) | 7 (50) | 18 (54) |
| Outborn, n (%) | 17 (90) | 12 (86) | 29 (88) |
| Apgar score at 5 min of ⩽ 5, n (%) | 12 (67) | 11 (79) | 23 (72) |
| Cord pH, mean (range) (group A, N = 12; group B, N = 11) | 6.87 (6.67–7.00) | 6.88 (6.64–7.30) | 6.87 (6.64–7.30) |
| Lactate level, mean (range), mmol/L (group A, N = 15; group B, N = 13) | 14.1 (2.2–26) | 9.3 (3.1–29.0) | 11.9 (2.2–29.0) |
| HIE, n (%) | | | |
| Grade II | 11 (58) | 7 (50) | 18 (55) |
| Grade III | 8 (42) | 7 (50) | 15 (45) |
| Mode of delivery, n (%) | | | |
| Vaginal | 3 (16) | 4 (29) | 7 (21) |
| Ventouse extraction | 2 (10) | 3 (21) | 5 (15) |
| Cesarean section, emergency | 14 (74) | 7 (50) | 21 (64) |
| Meconium-stained liquor, n (%) | 9 (47) | 7 (50) | 16 (49) |
| Mechanical ventilation, n (%) | 15 (79) | 13 (93) | 28 (85) |

## Duration of seizure patterns

For the 33 infants, we calculated a total duration of seizure patterns of 19,378 minutes (10.8 per cent of total registration time). For 12 of the 33 infants, there was ⩾ 1 episode of disagreement between the 2 reviewers regarding seizure discharges, but consensus was reached in all cases.

In both groups, there was a wide distribution of seizure discharges (Fig. 2). The duration (median ± SD) of seizure patterns was 196 ± 340 minutes in group A, compared with 503 ± 1,084 minutes in group B (Fig. 3). No significant difference in duration was found between the groups by using linear regression. In both groups, a longer duration of seizure activity was noted for infants with grade III HIE compared with infants with grade II HIE, although this difference was not significant ($P = .8$) (Fig. 4).

## AED treatment

Twelve infants (63 per cent) in group A and 9 infants (64 per cent) in group B received phenobarbitone in the referral hospital (given for treatment of suspected clinical seizures and not as prophylaxis). Fourteen (74 per cent) of the 19 infants in group A received ⩾ 3 AEDs, compared with 7 infants (50 per cent) in group B. These differences were not statistically significant.

## aEEG analysis and AED treatment in group A

In a review of data for the 19 infants in group A, treatment was appropriate for only 8 infants. For the other 11 infants, seizures existed for ⩾ 2 hours before treatment was started or a second- or third-line AED was given or treatment was not effective but no other AED was given. In a

Table 4. aEEG characteristics

| | Group A (N = 19) | Group B (N = 14) | Total (N = 33) |
|---|---|---|---|
| Start of aEEG registration, median (range), h after birth | 4.5 (2–23) | 6.5 (0.5–24) | 5 (0.5–24) |
| Start of clinical seizures, median (range), h after birth | 6.5 (1–22) | 3 (1–16) | 4.5 (1–22) |
| Start of randomization, median (range), h after birth | 15.25 (4–35) | 17.5 (5–31) | 16.75 (4–35) |
| Total monitoring time, median (range), h | 86.25 (10–170) | 87.75 (22–202.75) | 87 (10–202.75) |
| Background pattern before randomization, n (%) Continuous/discontinuous normal voltage Burst suppression Continuous low voltage/flat trace | 9 (48) 5 (26) 5 (26) | 3 (21) 4 (29) 7 (50) | 12 (36) 9 (28) 12 (36) |
| EEG status epilepticus, n (%) | 12 (63) | 10 (71) | 22 (67) |
| Given AED before monitoring, n (%) | 12 (63) | 9 (64) | 21 (64) |
| Total no. of AEDs administered, n (%) < 3 ⩾ 3 | 5 (26) 14 (74) | 7 (50) 7 (50) | 12 (36) 21 (64) |

comparison of the duration of seizure patterns for the infants who were treated appropriately ($n = 8$) and those who were not ($n = 11$), we found a significant difference in duration (37 vs. 248 minutes ($P = .02$).

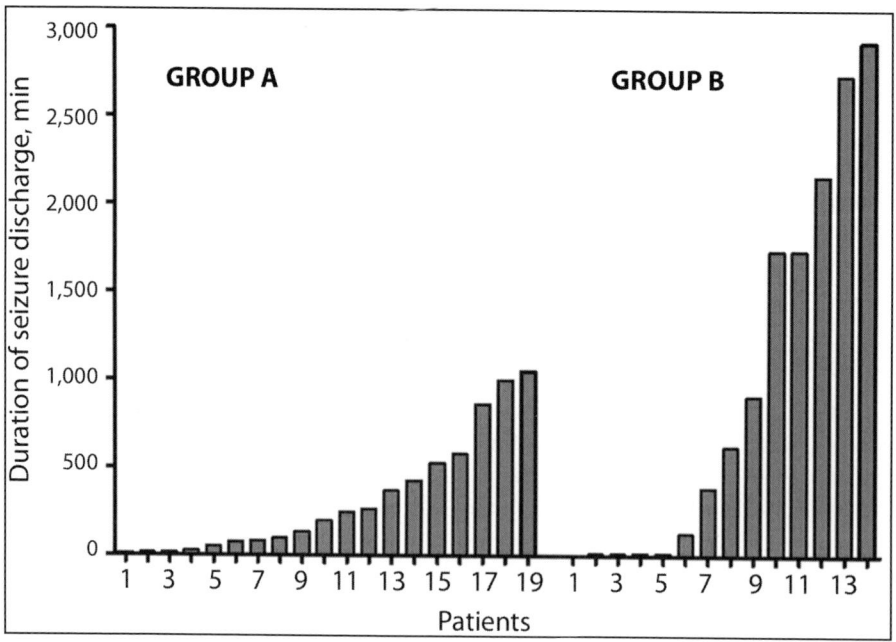

Fig. 2. Difference in distributions of total duration of seizure patterns in the treatment group (A) and the nontreatment group (B).

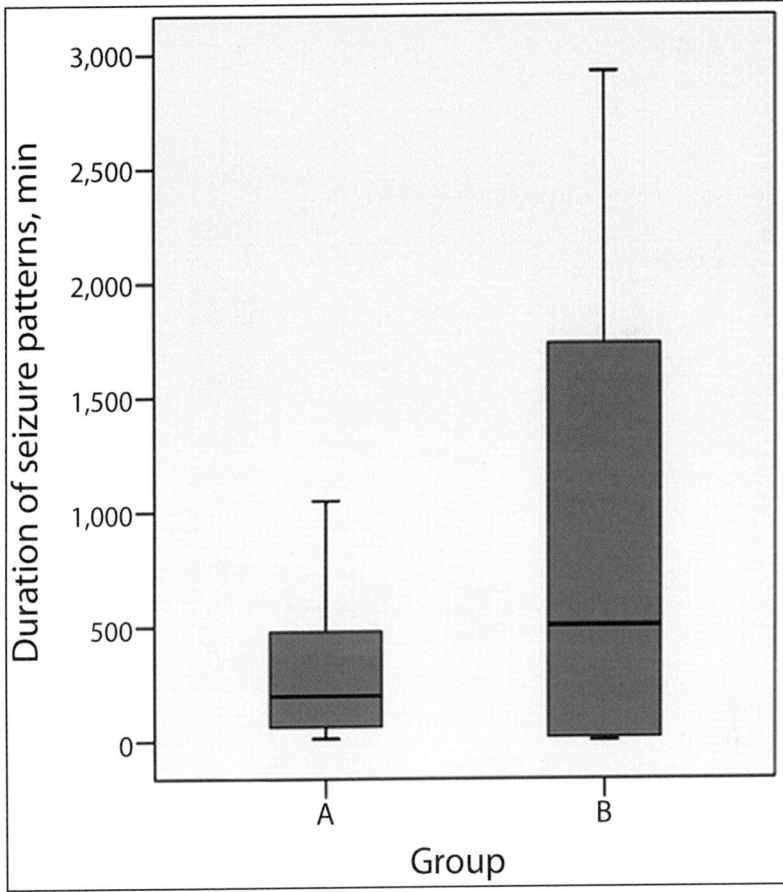

*Fig. 3. Box plot of duration of seizure patterns for the clinical and subclinical seizure treatment group (A) and the clinical seizure treatment group (B). The horizontal lines indicate the median; box, 25th and 75th percentiles. The vertical lines indicate the limit lines and the ranges.*

### aEEG analysis and AED treatment in group B

In a review of aEEG registration for the infants in group B, clinically suspected seizures (treated with 1 or 2 AEDs) could not be confirmed with aEEG for 6 of the 14 infants. All infants showed EEG seizure patterns several hours before ($n = 3$) or after ($n = 3$) treatment of clinically suspected seizures. For 7 infants, clinical manifestations were confirmed with aEEG. For 4 of those infants, seizure patterns existed for a longer time before clinical signs were seen; for 5 of them, clinical symptoms resolved after AED administration but EEG seizure patterns persisted. One infant, who was assigned randomly after a subclinical seizure pattern was observed, received no AEDs. No clinical signs were noted after blinding of the registration, and no new EEG seizures were seen in a review of the recording.

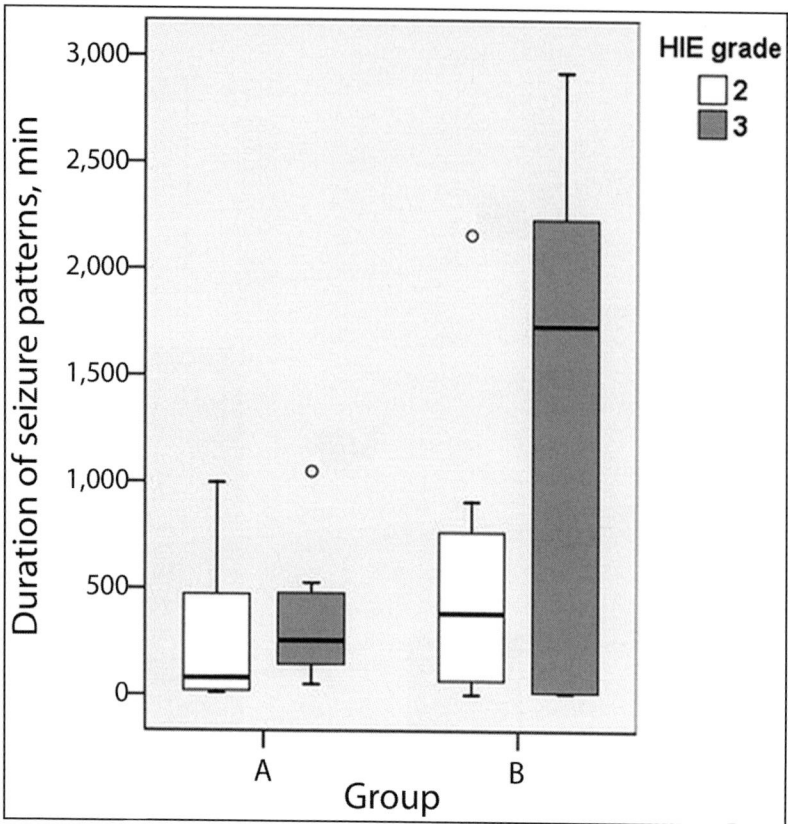

*Fig. 4. Box plot of duration of seizure patterns with respect to grade of HIE in group A and group B. The horizontal lines indicate the median; box, 25$^{th}$ and 75$^{th}$ percentiles. The vertical lines indicate the limit and the ranges.*

**MRI scores**

MRI was performed for 26 (79 per cent) of the 33 infants (15 in group A and 11 in group B). Infants in both groups underwent MRI at a mean age of 5.5 days (range: 3–9 days). We excluded 1 infant with bilateral perinatal arterial stroke from the analysis. In both groups, the median MRI score was 4. Five infants in group A and 4 in group B had MRI scores of < 4. When data for the whole group of 25 infants were assessed, there was a significant relationship between the duration of seizure patterns and MRI scores in linear regression analyses (Fig. 5). When analyses were performed for both groups, a significant relationship was found only in the blinded group (Fig. 5).

**Neonatal death**

Thirteen infants died during the neonatal period, including 6 in group A and 7 in group B. All except 1 infant had grade III HIE; for most of the infants, intensive care treatment was withdrawn because of an expected poor prognosis. This decision was based on multiple examinations, including clinical assessment, EEG background patterns and persistence of seizure patterns, and neuroimaging data (cranial ultrasound and/or MRI data). Infants who died during the neonatal period had a longer duration of seizure patterns than did than did survivors (428 vs. 164 minutes). Infants who died had shorter recording times because of withdrawal of intensive care, which probably restricted the total duration of seizure patterns. In the group of survivors, no significant differences between the groups with respect to time on a ventilator, time of stay in the NICU, and time to discharge were found.

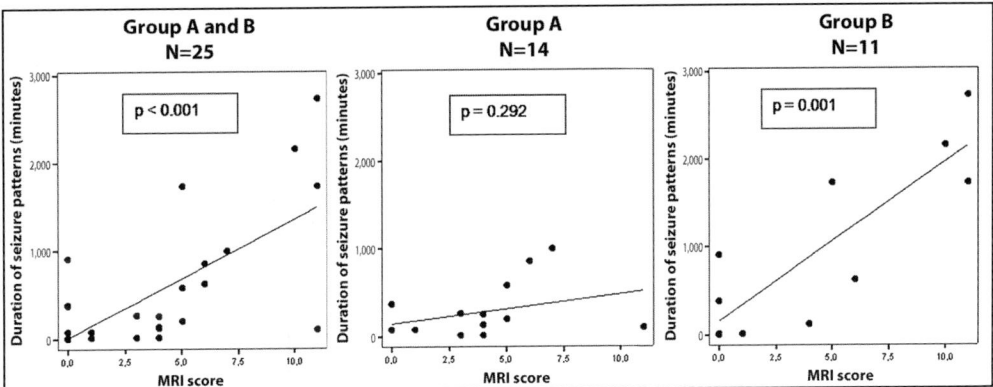

*Fig. 5. Relationship between duration of seizure patterns and MRI scores (linear regression).*

## Discussion

This is the first randomized, controlled trial studying the effect of treatment of subclinical seizures. In this small group of infants, we found a trend for reduction of seizure duration when clinical and subclinical seizure patterns detected with aEEG were treated, although this trend was not statistically significant.

There was no statistically significant difference between groups in the number of AEDs used, although 74 per cent of the infants in the active treatment group received ⩾ 3 drugs, compared with 50 per cent in the other group (treatment of clinical seizures only). It was noted that infants who were treated appropriately for both clinical and subclinical seizure patterns received more AEDs within a relatively short period, which resulted in a significantly shorter duration of seizure patterns, compared with those who were not treated appropriately. This suggests that treatment is more likely to be effective when it is initiated without delay. It is possible that the differences between groups would have been stronger and perhaps even statistically significant if treatment of the infants in the active treatment group had been optimal for all infants.

The mortality rate was lower in group A (32 per cent) than in group B (50 per cent). Although the 2-year assessment of the infants is still awaited, MRI results now are often considered as markers for short-term outcomes. A significant association was found between seizure pattern duration and higher MRI scores (more-severe brain injury), especially for infants in the blinded group who had a longer duration of seizure patterns. This finding supports the assumption that prolonged clinical and subclinical seizures induce or enhance already-existing brain injury (McBride *et al.*, 2000; Miller *et al.*, 2002; Wirrell *et al.*, 2001). Wirrell *et al.* (2001) reported that seizures superimposed on hypoxic ischaemia significantly exacerbated brain injury in rat pups. Translation of these findings into clinical practice is complicated. In human studies, it is difficult to measure the effect of seizures on neuronal injury and to distinguish this from the underlying pathogenesis of brain damage and possible effects of AED treatment. The few available studies in neonates do suggest that seizures are likely to increase neuronal injury (Glass et al., 2009; Legido et al., 1991; McBride et al., 2000; Miller et al., 2002; van Rooij et al., 2007).

Only neonates with HIE were included in this study, to yield a homogeneous group. Only one infant also showed bilateral perinatal arterial stroke. The median duration of seizure patterns in this group of infants with HIE was longer than expected. One half of the patients had grade II HIE and, because most of the infants were undergoing mechanical ventilation and showed some signs of multiorgan failure, it is likely that we included more-severely affected infants within the moderate HIE spectrum. All infants developed their first seizure and were admitted within 24 hours after birth. Infants with mild grade II HIE would by definition show clinical seizures (Sarnat & Sarnat, 1976).When their seizures were controlled with a loading dose of phenobarbitone and the infants were otherwise faring well, they usually would not be referred to a NICU and therefore would not be eligible for our study.

Four infants were excluded from analyses because they showed no EEG seizures retrospectively. Three of them were assigned randomly to group A. Only 2 of them received phenobarbitone in the referral hospital. In all cases, the suspected seizure discharge was restricted to a single short episode and the decision was made not to treat the infants. All 4 infants showed normal background patterns and survived the neonatal period.

Our study is an aEEG study, and it is well recognized that this technique has limitations. Previous studies showed that short and focal seizures may be missed (Hellström-Westas, 1992; Toet et al., 2002). Shellhaas et al. (2007) reported that aEEG alone has significant limitations in the diagnosis and quantification of neonatal seizures. In that study, however, the interpreters had no access to the raw EEG data when evaluating aEEG recordings. New digital aEEG devices do have access to a simultaneous display of the original raw EEG signal, and a novel seizure-detection algorithm has been developed to improve seizure detection with aEEG (Navakatikyan et al., 2006; Shah et al., 2006, 2008; Shellhaas & Clancy, 2007). This probably will help to increase expertise in the recognition of seizures. For our study, we included only seizures that were confirmed by the raw 1-channel EEG tracing. In a recent study by Shah et al. (2008), 76 per cent of seizures seen on full cEEG recordings were identified by using 2-channel aEEG with access to the raw 2-channel EEG tracings. The long duration of the aEEG registration seems to outweigh the limitations of obtaining detailed information during a much shorter, 30-minute cEEG registration. aEEG does not replace cEEG, and $\geqslant 1$ cEEG study should be performed for every child presenting with moderate or severe encephalopathy.

A limitation of our study is the study population. Before the study was started, a sample size of 130 infants was calculated with power analysis. Obtaining informed parental consent was more difficult than anticipated, because the parents were reluctant to allow blinding of the monitoring device. Also, parents were asked to give permission shortly after an unexpected complicated delivery of a critically ill infant who required acute neonatal transfer to a level 3 NICU. Another limitation is that we did not use video registration; therefore, we cannot exclude the possibility that some subclinical seizures had some subtle clinical symptoms (Murray et al., 2008; Volpe, 2001). However, Murray et al. (2008) showed that only 27 per cent of clinically suspected seizures were subsequently confirmed to be ictal discharges with cEEG. This was also seen in our study, because infants in group B were sometimes treated for clinical seizures that could not be confirmed with aEEG or EEG. These movements have been described as 'motor automatism' of uncertain origin (Mizrahi & Kellaway, 1987). One could imagine that these movements were indeed seizures but, being focal, were not identified with single-channel aEEG or EEG recording.

Furthermore, there was a discrepancy in the level of expertise at the participating centres, with 2 centres having > 10 years of experience and other centres having started using the technique only recently. This lack of experience probably led to a delay in seizure treatment of 11 infants in group A.

## Conclusions

We report the results of the first randomized, controlled trial of treatment of subclinical seizures. In this small group of infants with HIE, a trend was found for a reduction in the duration of seizure patterns when clinical seizures and subclinical seizure patterns were treated. This trend, as well as the significant association of seizure duration and severity of brain injury found on MRI scans, which was seen for infants who received treatment for clinical seizures only, suggests that recognition and treatment of neonatal seizures in infants with HIE can reduce brain injury.

**Acknowledgments:** Dr van Rooij was supported by the Dutch Epilepsy Foundation (Grant NEF 3–15).

## References

Barkovich, A.J., Hajnal, B.L., Vigneron, D., *et al.* (1998): Prediction of neuromotor outcome in perinatal asphyxia: evaluation of MR scoring systems. *AJNR Am. J. Neuroradiol.* **19**, 143–149.

Bittigau, P., Sifringer, M., Genz, K., *et al.* (2002): Antiepileptic drugs and apoptotic neurodegeneration in the developing brain. *Proc. Natl. Acad. Sci USA* **99**, 15089–15094.

Bittigau, P., Sifringer, M. & Ikonomidou, C. (2003): Anti-epileptic drugs and apoptosis in the developing brain. *Ann. N.Y. Acad. Sci.* **993**, 103–114.

Boylan, G.B., Rennie, J.M., Pressler, R.M., *et al.* (2002): Phenobarbitone, neonatal seizures, and video-EEG. *Arch. Dis. Child Fetal Neonatal Ed.* **86**, F165–F170.

Brunquell, P.J., Glennon, C.M., DiMario, F.J., Jr, Lerer, T. & Eisenfeld, L. (2002): Prediction of outcome based on clinical seizure type in newborn infants. *J. Pediatr.* **140**, 707–712.

Clancy, R.R. & Legido, A. (1991): Postnatal epilepsy after EEG-confirmed neonatal seizures. *Epilepsia* **32**, 69–76.

Clancy, R.R., Legido, A. & Lewis, D. (1988): Occult neonatal seizures. *Epilepsia* **29**, 256–261.

Glass, H.C., Glidden, D., Jeremy, R.J., Barkovich, A.J., Ferriero, D.M. & Miller, S.P. (2009): Clinical neonatal seizures are independently associated with outcome in infants at risk for hypoxic-ischaemic brain injury. *J. Pediatr.* **155**, 318–323.

Hellström-Westas, L. (1992): Comparison between tape-recorded and amplitude-integrated EEG monitoring in sick newborn infants. *Acta Paediatr.* **81**, 812–819.

Hellström-Westas, L. & Rosen, I. (2006): Continuous brain-function monitoring: state of the art in clinical practice. *Semin. Fetal Neonatal Med.* **11**, 503–511.

Hellström-Westas, L., Blennow, G., Lindroth, M., Rosen, I. & Svenningsen, N.W. (1995): Low risk of seizure recurrence after early withdrawal of antiepileptic treatment in the neonatal period. *Arch. Dis. Child Fetal Neonatal Ed.* **72**, F97–F101.

Lawrence, R., Mathur, A., Nguyen The Tich, S., Zempel, J. & Inder, T. (2009): A pilot study of continuous limited-channel aEEG in term infants with encephalopathy. *J. Pediatr.* **154**, 835–841.

Legido, A., Clancy, R.R. & Berman, P.H. (1991): Neurologic outcome after electro-encephalographically proven neonatal seizures. *Pediatrics* **88**, 583–596.

Levene, M. (2002): The clinical conundrum of neonatal seizures. *Arch. Dis. Child Fetal Neonatal. Ed.* **86**, F75–F77.

Malingré, M.M., van Rooij, L.G., Rademaker, C.M., *et al.* (2006): Development of an optimal lidocaine infusion strategy for neonatal seizures. *Eur. J. Pediatr.* **165**, 598–604.

McBride, M.C., Laroia, N. & Guillet, R. (2000): Electrographic seizures in neonates correlate with poor neurodevelopmental outcome. *Neurology* **55**, 506–513.

Miller, S.P., Weiss, J., Barnwell, A., et al. (2002): Seizure-associated brain injury in term newborns with perinatal asphyxia. *Neurology* **58,** 542–548.

Mizrahi, E.M. & Kellaway, P. (1987): Characterization and classification of neonatal seizures. *Neurology* **37,** 1837–1844.

Murray, D.M., Boylan, G.B., Ali, I., Ryan, C.A., Murphy, B.P. & Connolly, S. (2008): Defining the gap between electrographic seizure burden, clinical expression, and staff recognition of neonatal seizures. *Arch. Dis. Child Fetal Neonatal Ed.* **93,** F187–F191.

Navakatikyan, M.A., Colditz, P.B., Burke, C.J., et al. (2006): Seizure detection algorithm for neonates based on wave-sequence analysis. *Clin. Neurophysiol.* **117,** 1190–1203.

Rutherford, M.A., Pennock, J.M., Counsell, S.J., et al. (1998): Abnormal magnetic resonance signal in the internal capsule predicts poor neurodevelopmental outcome in infants with hypoxic-ischaemic encephalopathy. *Pediatrics* **102,** 323–328.

Sarnat, H.B. & Sarnat, M.S. (1976): Neonatal encephalopathy following fetal distress: a clinical and electroencephalographic study. *Arch. Neurol.* **33,** 696–705.

Shah, D.K., Lavery, S., Doyle, L.W., et al. (2006): Use of 2-channel bedside electroencephalogram monitoring in term-born encephalopathic infants related to cerebral injury defined by magnetic resonance imaging. *Pediatrics* **118,** 47–55.

Shah, D.K., Mackay, M.T., Lavery, S., et al. (2008): Accuracy of bedside electroencephalographic monitoring in comparison with simultaneous continuous conventional electroencephalography for seizure detection in term infants. *Pediatrics* **121,** 1146–1154.

Shellhaas, R.A. & Clancy, R.R. (2007): Characterization of neonatal seizures by conventional EEG and single-channel EEG. *Clin. Neurophysiol.* **118,** 2156–2161.

Shellhaas, R.A., Soaita, A.I. & Clancy, R.R. (2007): Sensitivity of amplitude-integrated electroencephalography for neonatal seizure detection. *Pediatrics* **120,** 770–777.

Scher, M.S., Painter, M.J., Bergman, I., Barmada, M.A. & Brunberg, J. (1989): EEG diagnoses of neonatal seizures: clinical correlations and outcome. *Pediatr. Neurol.* **5,** 17–24.

Scher, M.S., Alvin, J., Gaus, L., Minnigh, B. & Painter, M.J. (2003): Uncoupling of EEG-clinical neonatal seizures after antiepileptic drug use. *Pediatr. Neurol.* **28,** 277–280.

Sicca, F., Contaldo, A., Rey, E. & Dulac, O. (2000): Phenytoin administration in the newborn and infant. *Brain Dev.* **22,** 35–40.

Toet, M.C., van der Meij, W., de Vries, L.S., Uiterwaal, C.S.P.M. & van Huffelen, K.C. (2002): Comparison between simultaneously recorded amplitude integrated electroencephalogram (cerebral function monitor) and standard electroencephalogram in neonates. *Pediatrics* **109,** 772–779.

Toet, M.C., Groenendaal, F., Osredkar, D., van Huffelen, A.C. & de Vries, L.S. (2005): Postneonatal epilepsy following amplitude-integrated EEG-detected neonatal seizures. *Pediatr. Neurol.* **32,** 241–247.

van Rooij, L.G., de Vries, L.S., Handryastuti, S., et al. (2007): Neurodevelopmental outcome in term infants with status epilepticus detected with amplitude-integrated electroencephalography. *Pediatrics* **120,** 1202: e354–e363.

Volpe, J.J. (2001): *Neurology of the Newborn* (4$^{th}$ ed.) Philadelphia, PA: Saunders.

Wirrell, E.C., Armstrong, E.A., Osman, L.D. & Yager, J.Y. (2001): Prolonged seizures exacerbate perinatal hypoxic-ischaemic brain damage. *Pediatr. Res.* **50,** 445–454.

## Chapter 2

# Neurologic assessment and cerebral MRI in preterm infants

Licia Lugli, Isotta Guidotti, Natascia Bertoncelli and Fabrizio Ferrari

*Neonatology Unit, Modena University Hospital, via del Pozzo 71, 41100 Modena, Italy*
fabrizio.ferrari@unimore.it

## Summary

One major issue of neonatologists and developmental neurologists is to identify infants at risk for subsequent neurodevelopmental disability who may benefit from a strict neurologic follow-up and early intervention strategies.

Brain injury during the perinatal period is the most common cause of morbidity for preterm infants. These brain injuries include germinal matrix intraventricular haemorrhage, post-haemorrhagic hydrocephalus, and periventricular leucomalacia (PVL).

The presence of cystic PVL, which consists of focal necrotic lesions, evolving to cysts, is highly predictive of cerebral palsy. Diffuse noncystic white matter abnormalities (referred to as diffuse PVL or white matter abnormality [WMA]) have also been shown to be predictive of later neurodevelopmental impairments in very-preterm infants. Diffuse WMA is the most common brain abnormality found in preterm infants examined with MRI at term; it may be suspected on the basis of MRI signal change, and is often accompanied by ventricular dilatation and white matter atrophy.

A thorough neurologic assessment is mandatory for evaluating neurologic deficits and functional impairments due to the brain injury. Prechtl's method of assessing spontaneous movements in infants, known as assessment of general movements (GMs), is reported to have a higher predictive validity compared to both neurologic examination and cranial ultrasound as far as the long-term outcome of preterm infants is concerned. GM assessments have demonstrated a greater sensitivity in predicting CP than have other motor assessments that can be used in early infancy.

The combination of a functional assessment and a tool evaluating brain structure (MRI) may lead to greater accuracy in predicting those infants who are at risk of motor impairment.

## Introduction

Because of advances in perinatal medicine, survival rates for preterm infants have improved considerably, but preterm survivors nevertheless remain at risk for motor, cognitive, sensory, behavioural, and health problems (Marlow *et al.*, 2005).

One major issue for neonatologists and developmental neurologists is to identify those infants at risk for subsequent neurodevelopmental disability who may nonetheless benefit from rigorous neurologic follow-up and early-intervention strategies.

Brain injury during the perinatal period is the most common cause of morbidity for preterm infants. These brain injuries include germinal matrix intraventricular haemorrhage (GMH-IVH), post-haemorrhagic hydrocephalus, and periventricular leucomalacia (PVL).

The presence of cystic PVL, which consists of focal necrotic lesions, evolving to cysts, is highly predictive of cerebral palsy (CP). Diffuse noncystic white matter abnormalities (referred to as diffuse PVL or white matter abnormality [WMA]) have also been shown to be predictive of later neurodevelopmental impairments in very-preterm infants. Diffuse WMA is the most common brain abnormality found in preterm infants examined with MRI at term; it may be suspected on the basis of MRI signal change, and is often accompanied by ventricular dilatation and white matter atrophy. Such alterations have been shown to be poorly detected on cranial ultrasound, limiting the potential of cranial ultrasound in predicting outcomes. However, accessibility to MRI for some preterm infants is limited and it would be helpful to have functional assessment tools, available at the bedside and useful in prognostication (De Vries & Groenendaal, 2002).

A thorough neurologic assessment is mandatory for evaluating neurologic deficits and functional impairments due to the brain injury. Prechtl's method of assessing spontaneous movements in infants, known as assessment of general movements (GMs), is reported to have a higher predictive validity compared to both neurologic examination and cranial ultrasound as far as the long-term outcome of preterm infants is concerned. GM assessments have demonstrated a greater sensitivity in predicting CP than have other motor assessments that can be used in early infancy (Prechtl et al., 1997).

The combination of a functional assessment and a tool evaluating brain structure (MRI) may lead to greater accuracy in predicting those infants who are at risk of motor impairment.

## Poor outcome

Outcome in preterm births can be categorized into severe and moderate-to-mild deficits. Severe deficits comprise cerebral palsy, mental retardation (developmental quotient of less than 70), and severe visual or hearing impairment. Severe deficits can be detected within the first two years of life. Moderate-to-mild deficits, however, are often not detected until school age. Cerebral palsy (CP) is one of the major disabilities of preterm birth and is defined as a group of disorders of movement and postural control caused by a nonprogressive defect or lesion of the developing brain (Rosenbaum et al., 2005). The leading prenatal and perinatal risk factors for CP are birthweight and gestational age, but other risk factors include neonatal encephalopathy, pregnancy with multiple foetuses, infection and inflammation, and a variety of genetic factors (Marlow et al., 2005).

## Traditional neurologic examination

The traditional neurologic examination remains fundamental to identify, during the neonatal period and later on during the first two years of life, neurologic abnormalities (Dubowitz et al., 1998a; Volpe, 2008). A variety of standardized examination tools have been developed to estimate gestational age and to detect neurologic abnormalities and determine their course during development by repeated assessment. A widely used examination method is that of Dubowitz et al. (1998a). Normative data exist for different gestational age categories. Of importance, healthy preterm infants, when examined at term, are more hyperexcitable and tend to have less flexor tone in the limbs than do full-term infants. After discharge, preterm infants are included in a follow-up program, and serial neurologic examinations are performed during the first year of life with the aim of identifying early markers of abnormal neurologic development. A simple and scorable neurologic examination for infants between 2 and 24 months of age was developed in the Paediatric Department of the Hammersmith Hospital in London (the Infant Neurological Examination – HINE) (Haataja et al., 1999). This assessment consists of 37 items, divided into three sections: The first section includes 26 items evaluating cranial nerve function, posture, movements, tone and reflexes; the second section includes eight items evaluating the development of motor *function*; and the third section evaluates behaviour. It was standardized in a low-risk population of full-term infants assessed between 12 and 18 months of age, and an optimality score was developed on the basis of the frequency distribution of the findings for each item (Dubowitz et al., 1998b). The prognostic power of the HINE optimality score was recently explored in a population of very preterm infants between 9 and 18 months of age (Frisone et al., 2002). These authors found that 52 per cent of the premature cohort had optimal scores and 48 per cent had suboptimal scores. The magnitude of the scores was not significantly associated with the degree of prematurity, and by using an optimality score with an adjusted cut-off value, a very high sensitivity and specificity to predict walking at 2 years were shown. The scores were also not invariably associated with the pattern of ultrasonogram findings. Normal ultrasound tended to be associated with optimal scores and PVL with low scores, whereas other ultrasonogram abnormalities were associated with both optimal and suboptimal scores. This is not unexpected because haemorrhages and periventricular densities can be associated with both normal and abnormal neurodevelopment. This has demonstrated that a standardized neurologic examination performed as early as 9 months can be used reliably in very-preterm infants to predict motor outcome. The HINE was longitudinally performed at 3, 6, 9, and 12 months'-corrected age in a large population of preterm infants below 32 weeks' gestation: a high correlation, as early as 3 months onwards, between the HINE and the developmental quotient at 24 months was found (Romeo et al., 2009). This held true for both subscales of the developmental test used: the one assessing receptive and expressive language development and the one measuring visual-motor problem-solving skills. The high predictive value of the HINE across the first year of life was probably granted by the effective combination of different groups of items for each age period. Indeed, although a number of items were found to be consistently among the most predictive ones (movement quality and quantity and lateral tilting), other items changed across time. Tone items (ventral suspension, arm pronation/supination, and scarf sign), tended to be more predictive at 3 and 6 months post-term while maturational items, such as arm protection, vertical suspension, and forward parachute, were highly predictive only after 9 months. Cut-off values of optimality in very-preterm infants for the examinations at 3, 6, 9, and 12 months post-term were provided. A limited number of preterm infants (38 per cent) had optimal scores ($\geqslant 73$) at 12 months. The HINE scores were not strictly associated with the pattern of ultrasound scan (US) findings, as previously reported. Therefore, this study confirmed the high predictive value of neurologic examination in very preterm infants from 9 to 12 months post-term age, and extended it to examinations performed as early as 3 months post-term.

**Spontaneous movement patterns and general movements**

Prematurity is a condition associated with the highest risk of developing CP. Cerebral palsy occurs in 8 to 10 per cent of very-preterm infants, and approximately 40 per cent of all children with CP were born preterm. In preterm infants spastic diplegia prevails, followed by hemiplegia (Marlow et al., 2005).

An early prediction of CP will lead to strict neurologic follow-up study and to earlier enrollment in a rehabilitation program (Hadders-Algra, 2001). Unfortunately, reliable identification of CP in very young infants is extremely difficult and demands specific expertise. It is generally reported that CP cannot be diagnosed before several months after birth or even before 2 years of age. A so-called silent period, lasting up to few months, has also been claimed.

The neurologic symptoms observed in the first months after birth in preterm infants who will develop CP are neither sensitive nor specific enough to afford reliable prognosis. Irritability, abnormal finger posture, spontaneous Babinski reflex, weakness of the lower limbs, transient abnormalities of tone, and delay in achieving motor milestones are some of the neurologic signs that have been described in these high-risk preterm infants. All these signs may be encountered before the onset of CP or during transient dystonia, dissociated motor development, and other transient neurologic disturbances that vanish during the first or second year of life.

In the last two decades, a technique for assessing spontaneous motor activity has been introduced and evaluated, namely Prechtl's assessment of general movements (GMs) (Prechtl et al., 1997). This approach, based on the observation of the infant without direct physical examination, has proved to be a reliable and sensitive method in the neonatal period and early infancy for predicting normal and abnormal motor outcome, particularly CP (Ferrari et al., 2002). It requires video-recording of a few minutes of spontaneous motility and the off-line observation of the quality of GMs. Serial assessments of GMs from preterm birth up to 3 to 5 months post-term age define the developmental trajectory. The assessment based on a developmental trajectory predicts CP at a much earlier age than do other neurologic assessments (Prechtl et al., 1997).

Since the 1970s Prechtl and Hopkins (1986) focused their attention on the spontaneous movements of the foetus observed with ultrasound scans: they recognized that spontaneous movement could be distinguished in movements clearly constant in form and therefore easily recognizable every time they occur. Prechtl defined these sequences of movements as 'movement patterns'; with the aid of ultrasound he was able to recognize several foetal movement patterns such as startles, GMs, isolated limb movements, twitches, stretches, breathing movements, hiccup, yawn, head rotation, head flexion, sucking and swallowing, and others (Prechtl, 1989). These features emerge as early as 9 to 12 weeks postmenstrual age (PMA). It is striking that they look complex and differentiated right from their first appearance onward, showing hardly any change in form in the first weeks after birth, despite the profound changes in environmental conditions: the intrauterine or extrauterine environment seems to have very little influence on their form. Two of these movement patterns, stretches and yawns, are even maintained throughout life without changing their form. Surprisingly, local and isolated movements of the limbs appear 1 to 2 weeks earlier than GMs. They continue to be present during the whole preterm period and they are seen until 5 to 6 months post-term. The young nervous system of the foetus generates these movement patterns without being stimulated: they are endogenously generated and reflect the spontaneous activity of the brain (Prechtl & Hopkins, 1986).

The chance to observe and record (and eventually measure) endogenously generated brain activity is one of the dreams of neurobiologists. Prechtl's idea is that spontaneous movements are markers for brain impairment and brain dysfunction (Prechtl et al., 1997).

It is likely that GMs are produced by complex nervous networks, the so-called central pattern generators (CPGs) that are located in different parts and at various brain levels, especially in the higher parts of medulla and in the brainstem. Breathing, sucking, chewing, eye movements, swimming, crawling, and walking are other spontaneous motor activities that appear to be endogenously generated (*i.e.*, generated without any recognizable external stimulus); the combination of these motor activities varies according to the ongoing behavioural states. During state 2, irregular breathing, slow and rapid eye and body movements are fired by CPGs (from this, the term of 'active' or 'agitated' sleep; during state 1 (or quiet sleep), regular breathing and no eye or body movements reflect the different neural mechanisms that actively inhibit (or modulate in the case of respiration) these motor activities from higher cortical and subcortical structures. GMs as well as the other movement patterns are typical of states 2, 4, and 5. Startles that appear in state 1 are the exception to the rule.

General movements consist of movements that involve the whole body in a variable sequence of arm, leg, neck, and trunk movements. They wax and wane in intensity, force, and speed, and they have a gradual beginning and end. Rotations along the axis of the limbs and continual changes in the direction of movement make them fluent and elegant and create the impression of complexity and variability. Minor changes of their form can be recognized throughout the term: at preterm age, GMs are of larger amplitude and are often accompanied by lifting of the pelvis; at term age they are smaller in amplitude and show a writhing character that gradually disappears, while fidgety GMs emerge at 6 to 9 weeks post-term age.

Among the other movement patterns, the GMs are the most frequent, but also the most complex patterns; it is likely that their complexity makes them more vulnerable and therefore more sensitive to brain dysfunction.

Brain lesions affect quality rather than quantity of GMs, as demonstrated by various studies (Ferrari *et al.*, 1990). There is only one exception to this rule: severe perinatal asphyxia is accompanied by a transient phase of hypokinesis. Otherwise preterm and writhing GMs lose their character of fluency, variability, and complexity and have a poor repertoire or are cramped-synchronized or chaotic. Abnormal fidgety GMs are either exaggerated or absent.

Poor-repertoire GMs are the most common abnormality; variability in sequence is lost or poor. When abnormal GMs are followed by normal fidgety movements, a recovery from brain lesions and a normal outcome are expected. When the fidgety movements are lacking, on the contrary, cerebral palsy is very likely to occur. A cramped, synchronized character of GMs is also a severe GM abnormality: it is scored when all limb and trunk muscles contract and relax almost simultaneously. If this abnormal character persists for weeks and it is accompanied and/or followed by no fidgety movements, the development of a spastic form of cerebral palsy is predictable (Ferrari *et al.*, 2002; Prechtl *et al.*, 1997).

**Putative neural substrate of abnormal GMs**

Definitely abnormal GMs are specifically, but not exclusively related to lesions of the brain. Movement quality can be transiently affected by illness, and movement abnormalities can vanish or become more distinct with increasing age. The predictive value of GM quality varies with the age at which GMs are scored and with the type of outcome. Best prediction is achieved by a longitudinal series of GM assessments. Infants who persistently show definitely abnormal GMs have a high risk (70–85 per cent) for the development of CP, and infants who persistently show cramped-synchronized GMs invariably develop CP. The predictive value of a single GM assessment improves with increasing age, with the highest predictive value at fidgety age (Hadders-Algra, 2004; Prechtl *et al.*, 1997).

The clinical data indicate that abnormal GMs are related to brain lesions and/or brain dysfunction. An intriguing question is whether abnormal GMs can be attributed to specific dysfunctions of the young brain. As GM complexity and variability seem to be generated by the cortical subplate and mediated by the motor efferent connections of the subplate, abnormal GMs may be the result of damage or dysfunction of the subplate and/or its connections, which run through the periventricular white matter. Subplate and periventricular white matter injury are currently considered to be the dominant encephalopathy of preterm infants, as reported by Volpe et al. (2008). Previously, it was thought that the focal necrotic, cystic lesion of the PVL was the major neuropathologic abnormality of preterm infants. After more precise imaging techniques were introduced, it became clear that diffuse, noncystic white matter injury is much more common than cystic PVL. It occurs in 20–50 per cent of the preterm infants born prior to 34 weeks. Diffuse WMA is the result of diffuse damage of axons and oligodendrocytes, and it is also correlated with a decrease of cortical gray matter volume at term age (Hadders-Algra, 2004).

One of our studies (Ferrari et al., 1990) on brain lesions and quality of GMs in preterm infants revealed that the presence of substantial ventricular dilatation, which might be regarded as a sign of diffuse periventricular white matter damage, showed a strong correlation with the presence of definitely abnormal GMs at fidgety age and neurologic outcome.

The data of this study by Ferrari et al. (1990) and the study by Guzzetta et al. (2003) showed that abnormal GMs are related to periventricular white matter abnormalities and to damage of the subplate efferent connections. The high vulnerability of the subplate neurons to hypoxia–ischaemia at preterm suggests that direct subplate damage may play an additional role in the generation of abnormal GMs.

## Neuroimaging predictors of outcome

Two main imaging techniques have been used for the prediction of neurodevelopmental outcome in the neonatal period: ultrasound (US) and magnetic resonance imaging (MRI).

### Cerebral ultrasound

US is a simple bedside tool and, when used repeatedly, its sensitivity and specificity can be very high, especially in preterm infants. Lesions can be detected by US in the majority of infants born below 32 weeks PMA who develop CP. Intraventricular haemorrhage (IVH) grades III and IV, PVL, and focal infarctions are major cerebral lesions detected by US in the preterm population. Also, infants with an IVH grade I-II have an almost double risk of developing neurodevelopmental impairment at 20 months compared with those without any haemorrhage. The degree of milder US findings (PVL grade 1 or 2) and size of the corpus callosum are also related to neuromotor function in school-age children without CP (De Vries & Dubowitz, 1985). But diffuse white matter injury has been shown to be poorly detected on cranial ultrasound, limiting its potential in predicting outcome (De Vries & Groenendaal, 2002).

New techniques, such as those using transmastoidal access, have improved the representation of the cerebellum, a structure that can also be injured in very-low-birthweight (VLBW) infants. Cerebellar injuries may contribute to long-term neurocognitive disabilities, independent of associated supratentorial parenchymal lesions (Limperopoulos et al., 2007).

## MRI: abnormalities and outcome

Magnetic resonance imaging provides detailed information about the location and the extent of the brain lesions. MRI of the preterm infant is best done at term-equivalent age when the myelination of the posterior limb of the internal capsule may be used as predictor of motor outcome (Woodward et al., 2006).

In preterm infants, MRI has been used to detect diffuse white matter abnormalities [WMAs] and gray matter changes. Gray matter abnormalities are also associated with the same risks, but to a lesser extent than WMAs, which can be detected in more than 50 per cent of VLBW infants and are predictive of CP, psychomotor delay in early childhood, and neurosensory impairment. Recently, it has been shown that hypoxic ischaemic encephalopathy (HIE), typically described in full-term infants, can be observed in preterm infants as well. These infants have a high incidence of basal ganglia thalamus (BGT) and brainstem involvement, and the lesions are associated with significant mortality and neurologic morbidity (Volpe, 2008). Advanced MRI techniques – such as volumetry and morphometry, diffusion tensor imaging, and tractography – have been used to better determine the full spectrum of brain injury. In infants born preterm and examined at term, abnormalities in the cortex and deep nuclear structures were related to the degree of immaturity at birth and to concomitant WM injury. Volumetric changes in the sensorimotor, premotor, midtemporal, and parieto-occipital areas could be related to intellectual performance at school age. Recent findings indicate that the hippocampal volume can be reduced in preterm-born infants, and that it is associated with reduced working memory, and cognitive and motor performance at 2 years of age. However, the significance of subtle abnormalities detected on MRI regarding long-term functioning is not yet fully understood (Woodward et al., 2006).

## GMs and cerebral MRI

Cerebral abnormalities that are identified on MRI at term-equivalent age in very-preterm infants predict later neurodevelopmental outcomes, with moderate to severe white matter injury being associated with severe cognitive delay, psychomotor delay, CP, and neurosensory impairment (Woodward et al., 2006; Marlow et al., 2005). Since the quality of GMs is believed to be modulated by cerebral functioning, there may be a relationship between quality of GMs and cerebral abnormalities detected by MRI in the preterm infant.

A recent study by Inder et al. (2003) showed a significant relationship between GMs at 1 and 3 months and the nature and extent of cerebral WMAs at term-equivalent age in infants who were born very preterm. IVH and PVL also had a significant relationship with GMs at 1 and 3 months. Diffuse WMAs are the most common (12–53 per cent) abnormalities found on MRI in very-preterm infants; WMAs have been shown to relate to adverse motor outcomes at later ages, but alterations in motor functioning (GMs) are present much earlier, during infancy.

The nature and severity of cerebral WMAs seem to be related to the persistence of abnormal motor behaviour in the first 3 months of life, as assessed by GMs, suggesting that cerebral white matter is the major neuropathology responsible for such early functional motor abnormalities. In contrast, no relationship has been found between GMs at 1 and 3 months and to qualitative gray matter disturbance seen on MRI. Both MRI and GM assessments are useful in delineating both cerebral structure and motor functioning in infants born preterm. Abnormality in GMs is likely to be related to underlying WMAs, and both evaluations may assist in selecting infants at risk for referral to early-intervention services (Spittle et al., 2008).

Perinatal clinical variables have been shown to be poorly predictive of long-term neurodevelopmental outcomes; therefore, combining functional, easy, economical GM assessments, which may be repeated through early infancy, with structural MRI in high-risk infants is reasonable.

In the study by Spittle *et al.* (2009), both WMA assessed by MRI at term and GM assessments at 1 and 3 months' corrected age were associated with motor function at 12 months' corrected age for infants born very preterm. However, all assessments have some limitations in predicting motor development at 12 months' corrected age, with no test having 100 per cent accuracy. WMAs had the greatest specificity (94–96 per cent) of all assessments, and although the sensitivity of WMAs was very good for detecting CP, the sensitivity for detecting motor dysfunction other than CP was low. GMs at 1 month had good sensitivity in detecting motor dysfunction at 12 months' corrected age, but it resulted in a large number of false-positive results. GMs at 3 months had better specificity for predicting CP, but the sensitivity was lower in a similar fashion to that of MRI. Although WMAs seen on MRI at term may have the greatest accuracy in predicting motor dysfunction at 12 months' corrected age, it may not be easily accessible to some very preterm infants; GMs therefore seem to have a high predictive value. WMAs and GMs both have a role in the early assessment of the very-preterm infants' development. It is important to note that no test has 100 per cent accuracy because of the influence of social, environmental, and biological factors on development. As reported above, several studies have demonstrated that GMs are related to cerebral injury, but it is still unclear whether alterations in regional cerebral development are related to these abnormal movements. In a recent study, it was hypothesized that abnormal GMs would be related to the brain metric measurements of the primary motor areas, namely the transverse diameter of the cerebellum and biparietal lobe: reduced cerebellar, biparietal, and bifrontal diameters and larger lateral ventricles were all predictive of abnormal GMs at 3 months, and in particular a reduced cerebellar diameter was predictive of abnormal GMs in addition to moderate to severe white matter abnormality and IVH (Spittle *et al.*, 2010).

Cerebellar injury is increasingly recognized as a problem in preterm infants; however, the significance of reduced cerebellar volumes in the preterm population and subsequent neurodevelopment is less clear. The reduction in cerebellar diameter at term has been shown to be predictive of later motor problems at 3 months' corrected age (Spittle *et al.*, 2010). In this study by Spittle *et al.* (2010), infants with reduced cerebellar volumes were found to be at increased risk of abnormal GMs at 3 months, even when white matter abnormality and IVH were accounted for, supporting a primary link between the cerebellum and GM quality for very-preterm infants. These findings suggest that the cerebellum plays an important role in motor function in very-preterm infants, although further research to support this hypothesis is needed.

Future research directions include detailed motor assessments and correlation with findings on advanced brain imaging techniques such as diffusion-weighted images, tractography, and neurovascular changes on functional MRI.

## Conclusions

The assessment of the quality of GMs has become one of the clinical tools used to evaluate the integrity of the young nervous system. It has been hypothesized that movement complexity is generated by the cortical subplate and that abnormal GMs are the result of damage or dysfunction of the subplate and its motor efferent connections in the periventricular white matter.

Early assessment of the severity and type of motor impairment is needed in order to counsel parents, provide ameliorating follow-up services, and allocate early-intervention programs. GM assessment, neurologic examination, psychomotor development, and neuroimaging evaluation are valuable and complementary tools for predicting outcome.

## References

De Vries, L. & Dubowitz, L.M. (1985): Cystic leucomalacia in preterm infant: site of lesion in relation to prognosis. *Lancet* **2**, 1075–1076.

De Vries, L. & Groenendaal, F. (2002): Neuroimaging in the preterm infant. *Ment. Retard. Dev. Disabil. Res. Rev.* **8**, 273–280.

Dubowitz, L., Dubowitz, V. & Mercuri, E. (1998a): The neurological assessment of the preterm and full-term newborn infant. In: *Clinics in developmental medicine,* 2nd ed., publication 18. London, UK: Mac Keith Press.

Dubowitz, L., Mercuri, E. & Dubowitz, V. (1998b): An optimality score for the neurologic examination of the term newborn. *J. Pediatr.* **133**, 406–416.

Ferrari, F., Cioni, G., Einspieler, C., Roversi, M.F., Bos, A.F., Paolicelli, P.B., et al. (2002): Cramped synchronized general movements in preterm infants as an early marker for cerebral palsy. *Arch. Pediatr. Adolesc. Med.* **156**, 460–467.

Ferrari, F., Cioni, G. & Prechtl, H.F. (1990): Qualitative changes of general movements in preterm infants with brain lesions. *Early Hum. Dev.* **23**, 193–231.

Frisone, M.F., Mercuri, E., Laroche, S., Fogliam, C., Maalouf, E.F., Haataja, L., et al. (2002): Prognostic value of the neurologic optimality score at 9 and 18 months in preterm infants born before 31 weeks' gestation. *J. Pediatr.* **140**, 57–60.

Guzzetta, A., Mercuri, E., Rapisardi, G., Ferrari, F., Roversi, M.F., Cowan, F., et al. (2003): General movements detect early signs of hemiplegia in term infants with neonatal cerebral infarction. *Neuropediatrics* **34**, 61–66.

Haataja, L., Mercuri, E., Regev, R., Cowan, M., Rutherford, M. & Dubowitz, V. (1999): Optimality score for the neurologic examination of the infant at 12 and 18 months of age. *J. Pediatr.* **135** (2 Pt 1) 153–161.

Hadders-Algra, M. (2001): Early brain damage and the development of motor behavior in children: clues for therapeutic intervention? *Neural Plast.* **8**, 31–49.

Hadders-Algra, M. (2004): General movements: a window for early identification of children at high risk for developmental disorders. *J. Pediatr.* **145**, S12–18.

Inder, T.E., Wells, S.J., Mogridge, N.B., Spencer, C. & Volpe, J.J. (2003): Defining the nature of the cerebral abnormalities in the premature infant: a qualitative magnetic resonance imaging study. *J. Pediatr.* **143**, 171–179.

Limperopoulos, C., Bassan, H. & Gauvreau, K. (2007): Does cerebellar injury in premature infants contribute to the high prevalence of long-term cognitive, learning, and behavioral disability in survivors? *Pediatrics* **120**, 584–593.

Marlow, N., Wolke, D., Bracewell, M.A., Samara, M. & EPICure Study Group (2005): Neurologic and developmental disability at six years of age after extremely preterm birth. *N. Engl. J. Med.* **352**, 9–19.

Prechtl, H.F. (1989): Fetal behaviour. *Eur. J. Obstet. Gynecol. Reprod. Biol.* **1**, 32.

Prechtl, H.F. & Hopkins, B. (1986): Developmental transformations of spontaneous movements in early infancy. *Early Hum. Dev.* **14**, 233–238.

Prechtl, H.F., Einspieler, C., Cioni, G., Bos, A.F., Ferrari, F. & Sontheimer, D. (1997): An early marker for neurological deficits after perinatal brain lesions. *Lancet* **349**, 1361–1363.

Romeo, D.M., Cioni, M., Scoto, M., Pizzardi, A., Romeo, M.G. & Guzzetta, A (2009): Prognostic value of a scorable neurological examination from 3 to 12 months post-term age in very preterm infants: a longitudinal study. *Early Hum. Dev.* **85**, 405–408.

Rosenbaum, P., Dan, B., Leviton, A., Paneth, N., Jacobsson, B. & Goldstein, M. (2005): The definition of cerebral palsy. In: *Proposed definition and classification of cerebral palsy,* eds. M. Bax, M. Goldstein, P. Rosenbaum et al. *Dev. Med. Child. Neurol.* **47**, 571–576.

Spittle, A.J., Brown, N.C., Doyle, L.W., Boyd, R.N., Hunt, R.W. & Bear, M. (2008): Quality of general movements is related to white matter pathology in very preterm infants. *Pediatrics* **121**, e1184–1189.

Spittle, A.J., Boyd, R.N., Inder, T.E. & Doyle, L.W. (2009): Predicting motor development in very preterm infants at 12 months' corrected age: the role of qualitative magnetic resonance imaging and general movements assessments. *Pediatrics* **123**, 512–517.

Spittle, A.J., Doyle, L.W., Anderson, P.J., Inder, T.E., Lee, K.J., Boyd, R.N. & Cheong, J.L.Y. (2010): Reduced cerebellar diameter in very preterm infants with abnormal general movements. *Early Hum. Dev.* **86,** 1–5.

Volpe, J.J. (2008): *Neurology of the Newborn*, 5th ed. Philadelphia: Saunders.

Woodward, L.J., Anderson, P.J., Austin, N.C., Howard, K. & Inder, T.E. (2006): Neonatal MRI to predict neurodevelopmental outcomes in preterm infants. *N. Engl. J. Med.* **355,** 685–694.

Chapter 3

# Neuroimaging techniques: general concepts

### Luca A. Ramenghi

*U.O. di Neonatologia Terapia Intensiva Neonatale Maggiore IRCCS, Fondazione 'Cà Granda' Policlinico,*
*via della Commenda 12, Milan, Italy*
luca.ramenghi@mangiagalli.it

## Summary

Transfontanellar cranial ultrasound remains a very important technique in daily practice, especially in studying the brain of very preterm and sick neonates treated in neonatal intensive care units, and its usefulness has been enhanced by the availability of magnetic resonance imaging (MRI). MRI allows the assessment of the developing brain throughout different gestational ages, can be used at appropriate term-age to observe *ex utero* morphologic maturation of the preterm brain, and can identify minor forms of white matter abnormalities of prematurity, such as punctuate lesions and diffuse excessive hyper signal intensities. Nevertheless, the value of MR imaging is fundamental in studying more mature babies, like late-preterm or at-term babies, especially when seizures occur, or to disclose signs of rare diseases such as venous thrombosis. In certain disorders, such as perinatal asphyxia, MRI is well able to predict prognosis even after the introduction of new forms of treatment like hypothermia.

## Introduction

Despite marked improvements in antenatal and perinatal care, perinatal brain injury remains one of the most important medical complications in the newborn, resulting in chronic handicapping conditions later in life.

The words *perinatal* and *brain damage* have often been associated not only in the medical literature, but also in scientific articles written for the layman. The life of the foetus and its neurologic integrity has always carried an implicit and reassuring meaning during all of pregnancy, yet the possibilities of investigating and diagnosing neurologic problems have only been able to be considered in recent years after the advent of prenatal ultrasound and pre- and neonatal MR. Therefore, before these advances became available, the only explanation given for later neurologic problems developing in infants was 'a difficult birth'.

Many years have passed since the introduction of transfontanellar cranial ultrasound (CUS) to diagnose acquired brain lesions in neonates, and CUS still remains a very important technique in the daily practice of neonatal units, but further improvements have been made thanks to the combination of different imaging modalities. MRI is the modality that allows the assessment of the developing brain in great detail because of its resolving power and its noninvasiveness in the absence of irradiation: Magnetic resonance techniques are unique in that they provide not only detailed structural, but also metabolic and functional information without the use of ionizing radiation. Conventional MRI is therefore now widely used for identifying normal and pathologic brain morphology, giving objective information about the structure of the neonatal brain during development and in the case of injury. Further advancement of MR techniques have revealed many unknown aspects of brain development and help to further characterize injury to the developing brain (Ramenghi & Hüppi, 2009; Ramenghi *et al.*, 2005; Rutherford, 2001).

## Application of imaging modalities

Imaging plays an important role in screening for congenital malformations and other significant intracranial abnormalities in infants with clinical suspicion of an underlying neurologic disorder. A growing number of babies undergo imaging investigations to confirm or to ameliorate a diagnosis initiated during fetal life; this is particularly true for babies who underwent fetal MRI.

In addition to imaging's ability to make a specific and recognizable diagnosis of a brain lesion, a particularly well-developed function of neuroimaging has been *prediction* of long-term outcome, especially after the introduction of magnetic resonance imaging (Ramenghi & Hüppi, 2009; Ramenghi *et al.*, 2005; Rutherford, 2001).

The imaging correlates for motor impairments are well recognized (cavitations in the periventricular white matter for premature infants, lack of normal visualization of posterior limbs of internal capsule), but as yet there is no imaging correlate for the neurocognitive and neurobehavioural disorders that frequently develop in children born preterm (Bassi *et al.*, 2008).

While diffusion-weighted imaging provides most clinical benefit by identifying areas of ischemia, it may also be used to characterize brain development in the preterm infant without lesions. The clinical significance of preterm lesions, such as periventricular leucomalacia and haemorrhagic venous infarction, can be fully appreciated, the former giving rise to a spastic diplegia and the latter to a hemiplegia in those where the infarct involves the corticospinal tracts. We know that there is a lack of imaging correlates for neurocognitive disorders that frequently develop in children born preterm; however, MRI techniques may allow us to detect abnormalities responsible for these non-motor impairments, especially when associated with functional tests such as those for vision (Bassi *et al.*, 2008).

Fast diffusion-weighted imaging has provided understanding of the formation of white matter tracts in health and disease. Quantification of the brain and its structures is providing an accurate comparison of the structural development of the brain in neonates born at term and the functional development of the child. (Counsell *et al.*, 2008) This may produce more accurate neuroimaging correlates for later neurocognitive disorders. Spectroscopy is providing new insights into metabolic processes in response to injury (Groenendaal *et al.*, 1994) Functional imaging is limited in the newborn, but may also throw light on the mechanisms involved in normal and abnormal neurologic functioning (Fransson *et al.*, 2007).

## Neuroimaging modalities in the term-born neonate

### Ultrasound

An initial investigation with CUS in newborn babies born after the $37^{th}$ week of gestation and presenting neurologic symptoms is always justified. The possibility that CUS will clearly depict a perinatally acquired brain lesion in babies born at term is not high, especially during the very acute phase of the disorder. CUS can directly diagnose a specific pathologic disorder such as arterial stroke in case of a large lesion or it can help to identify a brain lesion caused by an underlying disease, such as an intraventricular bleed or a posterior fossa haemorrhage caused by a traumatic birth or by venous thrombosis. The value of CUS during the acute phase of hypoxic–ischaemic encephalopathy is pretty limited; it relies on the possibility of excluding other lesions mimicking asphyxia (*e.g.*, malformations, major subarachnoid or subdural haemorrhage, or, more rarely, stroke) or to identify very severe lesions of basal ganglia becoming visible only few days after the asphyctic event (Ramenghi & Hüppi, 2009; Ramenghi *et al.*, 2005; Rutherford, 2001).

## Computed tomography

Computed tomography (CT) has been abandoned over the last few years. Even the use of CT to better identify fresh bleeding or calcification is easily performed by specific functions of magnetic resonance imaging such as T2*, also called paramagnetic imaging. CT remains useful in 3-dimensional applications to certify craniosynostosis.

## MRI in the symptomatic term newborn baby

Seizures remain a significant issue in the neonatal period because they represent the most distinctive sign of neurologic disorder. A seizure is a transient alteration in neurologic function involving motor activity, changes in level of alertness, and impairment in autonomic function. Determination of aetiology is crucial in planning specific treatment and in formulating the first prognostic statement. For this purpose it is useful to differentiate seizing babies born with a normal Apgar score from those very depressed at birth who are suffering from perinatal asphyxia. The most common causative conditions in the asphyctic group are focal brain lesions caused by hypoxia–ischaemia with typical distributions of lesions (basal ganglia and thalami, watershed areas, cortex), followed by arterial infarcts and haemorrhages. (Govaert *et al.*, 2009; Benders *et al.*, 2007) Central nervous system infections, transient metabolic disturbances like hypoglycaemia, congenital abnormalities of the brain including those due to chromosomal anomalies, inborn errors of metabolism and benign neonatal convulsions, familial and not, can also lead to neonatal seizures, and thus detailed neuroimaging is an important tool in the diagnostic work-up. Brain malformations can range from highly localized focal dysplasia not diagnosed with CUS to catastrophic defects partially diagnosed with CUS (Ramenghi & Hüppi, 2009).

In all circumstances of seizures occurring in term newborns, MRI is the ideal diagnostic neuroimaging tool. A clinical diagnostic suspicion has to rely on a careful medical history and on a statistical approach of the most likely causes; for instance, in case of sudden occurrence of seizures in a perfectly normal newborn, stroke and haemorrhage have to be excluded as a first hypothesis (Benders *et al.*, 2009).

## Understanding the different vulnerability of the brain

The recent exponential rise in detailed MR imaging studies has emphasized the concept of gestationally determined regional vulnerability in the brain: the site and nature of the injury sustained are determined by a combination of the characteristics of the insult, the specific tissue and cell vulnerability, and the gestation of the infant. The type of insult may also be partly dependent on gestation; for instance, acute perinatal hypoxic–ischaemic events characteristic in the term-born neonate presenting with hypoxic–ischaemic encephalopathy (HIE) may occur at earlier gestation periods, but such events occur less often in the infant born preterm with lesions developing in similar brain regions and in other areas characteristically more vulnerable in more-premature babies. Similarly to HIE for term babies, white matter lesions are considered the hallmark of injury to the preterm brain as they are characteristic of perinatal injury relating to inflammation, infection, or hypoglycaemia in the term brain, occurring in a small percentage of neonates with encephalopathy (Fig. 1) (Burns *et al.*, 2008; Rutherford *et al.*, 2010).

## Ultrasound in the brain of infants born preterm

Cranial ultrasound is usually performed through the anterior fontanel, which acts as an acoustic window. Directly after birth the fontanel may be very small on account of moulding of the sutures, and this may limit the visualization of the intracranial anatomy. The anterior fontanel remains open for much of the first year of life and begins to close at about 9 months, although as the infant grows, the scalp tissues thicken and detailed imaging of the infant brain gradually becomes more difficult. The posterior fontanel can also be used as an acoustic window, particularly to examine the posterior periventricular white matter and the occipital horns of the lateral ventricles. Taylor has described the advantages of scanning through the mastoid fontanel for evaluation of the cerebellum and brain stem and has suggested that these views should be routinely incorporated into the standard brain imaging protocol (Ramenghi & Hüppi, 2009; Ramenghi *et al.*, 2005). Scanning through the thin squamous temporal bone may be useful in certain clinical situations, particularly for Doppler assessment of the middle cerebral artery and branches of the circle of Willis. The transtemporal and the mastoid approaches also provide an axial view of the brain comparable with CT images and permit better visualization of the peripheral regions of the parietal lobes, which are often not well visualized through the anterior fontanel.

An ultrasound scanner for use in the neonatal unit should be easily maneuverable, have a good range of transducers to image both the extremely premature and the term infant, and have facilities for image documentation, including video recording and hardcopy images. Both grayscale and color Doppler imaging should be available; in the future, power Doppler imaging may become an important asset. The choice of transducer frequency is a compromise between resolution and penetration; high-frequency transducers give better resolution, but may have relatively poor penetration. In general 7–10-MHz sector transducers are appropriate for scanning the brain of the very preterm infant, whereas a 5-MHz transducer will be more appropriate for the infant born at term. Even lower frequency (*e.g.*, a 3.5-MHz transducer) may be necessary to adequately visualize the posterior fossa in an older infant. High-frequency (*e.g.* 10 MHz) linear or curved

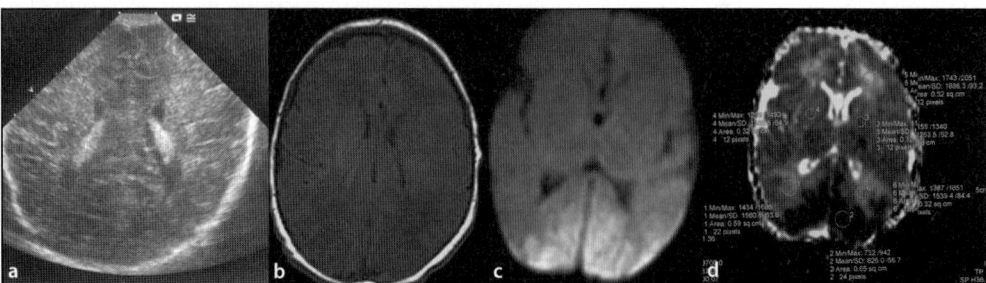

Fig. 1. Neuroimaging performed 2 hours after the onset of a severe hypoglycaemic event. **a.** coronal CUS; **b.** MR axial T1; **c.** MR axial DWI; **d.** MR axial apparent diffusion coefficient (ADC) map. US and conventional T1 imaging do not show any abnormality compared to those seen on DWI and ADC map, which show, respectively, reduction and pathologically low ADC values in the posterior areas of the brain.

linear transducers are particularly valuable to examine the posterior fossa through posterior access or extra-axial space, and the peripheral cerebral cortex immediately below the fontanel, which can be useful for evaluation of the superior sagittal sinus in conjunction with color Doppler imaging brain (Ramenghi & Hüppi, 2009).

Image acquisition and interpretation in ultrasound is operator-dependent and subject to interobserver error. It is crucial when performing any ultrasound examination to be meticulous with the gain settings to ensure that areas of altered echogenicity are not simply due to artifact. Scanning off-center through the anterior fontanelle may give rise erroneously to the impression of unilateral increased echodensity in the parenchyma. Similarly, misdiagnosis of transient echodensity may be made if the gain settings are too high or the slope of the time-gain compensation (TGC) is inappropriate. Conversely, abnormality may be overlooked when the gain is too low. It is important to ensure that the focus is set at an appropriate level which may need to be altered during the scanning sequence to examine both the periventricular regions and the structures of the posterior fossa. Subtle findings, such as mild echodensity, may not be easily reproduced on hard-copy images, which may pose a particular problem when the images are reported by radiologists and clinicians who have not performed the examination (Ramenghi & Hüppi, 2009; Ramenghi *et al.*, 2005; Rutherford, 2001).

## MRI in preterm babies

Magnetic resonance imaging is still a relatively new technique for imaging the very preterm infant. Any new developments in imaging the preterm infant have to be safe and quick, as time is of the essence when imaging a sick preterm infant. Fast diffusion-weighted imaging may increase our understanding of the formation of white matter tracts in health and disease. Quantification of the brain and its structures will allow us to accurately compare the development of the brain with the development of the child. This may produce more accurate neuroimaging correlates for later neurocognitive disorders (Fig. 2). Spectroscopy is providing new insights into metabolic processes in response to injury. Functional imaging is limited in the neonate, but may also shed light on the mechanisms involved in normal and abnormal neurologic functioning. The interpretation of images is greatly aided by accurate histologic comparisons, although it is becoming increasingly difficult to obtain consent for postmortem examination with retention of the brain (Ramenghi & Hüppi, 2009; Ramenghi *et al.*, 2005).

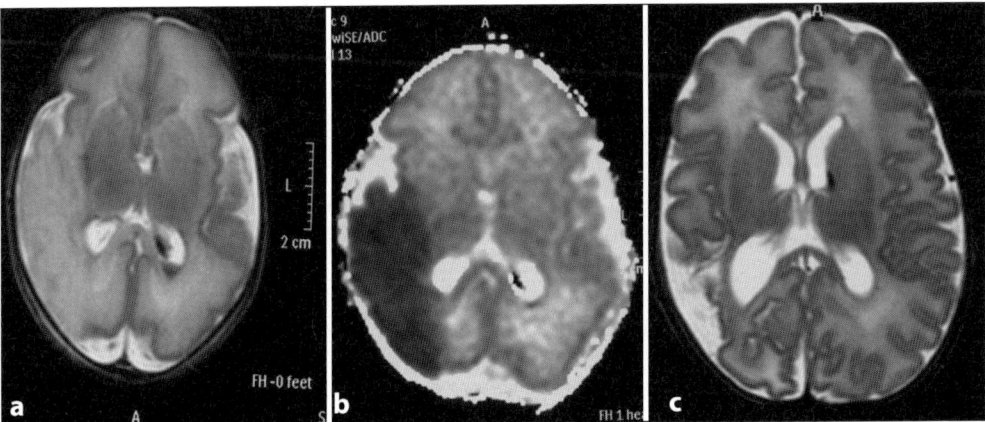

*Fig. 2.* ***a.*** *MR axial T2 and* (***b***) *MR axial ADC map in a 30-week-old preterm baby at 4 days of age showing the abnormal neuroimaging highly suggestive of a right arterial infarct (on T2 there is a loss of cortical detail and a more obvious reduction in apparent diffusion coefficient values). At term corrected age (****c****) the resulting infarcted area was smaller. At 5 years of age the child has left hemiplegia with good independent walking. At 2 years of age the child had been treated for recurrent seizures, but 18 months later was off medications.*

## MRI in the white matter of disease of prematurity

Periventricular leucomalacia (PVL) and parenchymal venous infarction complicating germinal matrix/intraventricular haemorrhage have long been recognized as the two significant white matter diseases responsible for the majority of cases of cerebral palsy in survivors of preterm birth. However, more recent studies using magnetic resonance imaging (MRI) to assess the preterm brain have documented two new appearances, adding to the spectrum of white matter disease of prematurity: punctate white matter lesions, and diffuse excessive high-signal intensity (DEHSI). These appear to be more common than PVL, but less significant in terms of their impact on individual neurodevelopment. They may, however, be associated with later cognitive and behavioural disorders known to be common after preterm birth. It remains unclear whether PVL, punctate lesions, and DEHSI represent a continuum of disorders occurring as a result of similar injurious process to the developing white matter (Fig. 3) (Ramenghi & Hüppi, 2009; Ramenghi *et al.*, 2005, 2007; Rutherford *et al.*, 2010a, 2010b).

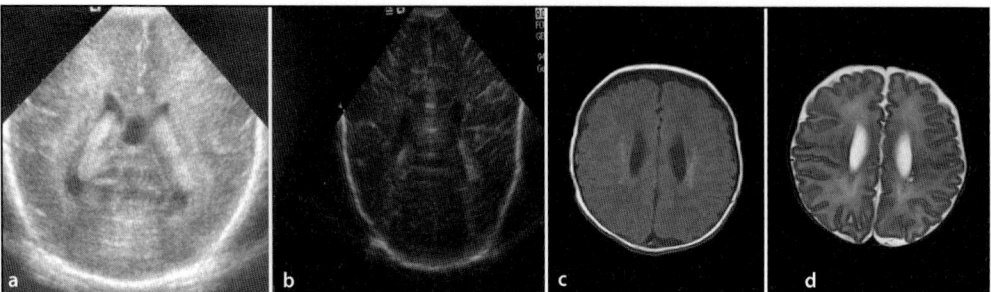

*Fig. 3.* **a.** *First CUS scan showing a persistently abnormal periventricular increased echogenicity at 10 days of a 29-week-old baby;* **b.** *US scan at term corrected age showed normal echogenicity, while MR axial T1 (**c**) and (**d**) T2 scans highlight periventricular abnormalities usually named 'punctate lesions'. On T1-weighted images these abnormalities at term corrected age can also represent mild glial scars.*

## Preterm brain at term

In some infants born prematurely there is ventricular dilation and widening of the extracerebral space at term, findings that suggest an incomplete maturation or a degree of cerebral atrophy. However, these findings may not be so clear on later follow-up imaging.

In some infants approaching term, the white matter develops a long T1, long T2 component, the so-called diffuse excessive high-signal intensity (DEHSI) on T2-weighted images. This is probably normal if restricted to the arrowheads and caps, but in some infants is more diffuse and extends beyond these areas towards the subcortical white matter. Infants with DEHSI show higher apparent diffusion coefficient (ADC) values on diffusion-weighted imaging (DWI) associated with the development of abnormally long T2, consistent with glial tissue, in the periventricular white matter at two years of age. These later changes could be described as a mild form of periventricular leucomalacia, but while they may be associated with ventricular dilation, the ventricular outline is usually abnormal. The corpus callosum may be thin. These periventricular and corpus callosal changes are a common finding when ex-preterm children and adolescents are imaged, but the exact relationship to later neurodevelopmental and neurocognitive deficits remains unclear. It is possible that these relatively focal changes are the visible side of a process that may have affected a much larger amount of developing brain, so-called perinatal teloleucoencehalopathy or white matter disease of prematurity (Ramenghi & Hüppi, 2009; Ramenghi *et al.*, 2005; Rutherford *et al.*, 2010b).

## Going beyond the picture

The association between structure and function in the developing brain deserves major attention. We have recently shown that probabilistic diffusion tractography provides quantitative information regarding white matter microstructure in the optic radiations in preterm infants at term-equivalent age and that fractional anisotropy (FA) correlates with visual assessment scores. Therefore, even at term-equivalent age, the maturation and integrity of optic radiations seems to be a major factor for the normal development of visual function.

Improvements in understanding very early and specific impairments in neurologic functions are important as the identification of early impairment will imply early enrollment in intervention programmes, which have been shown to influence favourably the developmental outcome of these infants. Understanding early human brain development is of great clinical importance, as many neurologic and neurobehavioural disorders have their origin in early structural and functional cerebral organization and maturation. Technological advances in neonatal brain imaging have made a major contribution to the understanding of disorders of the neonatal brain.

## References

Bassi, L., Ricci, D., Volzone, A., *et al.* (2008): Probabilistic diffusion tractography of the optic radiations and visual function in preterm infants at term equivalent age. *Brain* **131**, 573–582.

Benders, M.J., Groenendaal, F., Uiterwaal, C.S., *et al.* (2007): Maternal and infant characteristics associated with perinatal arterial stroke in the preterm infant. *Stroke* **38**, 1759–1765.

Benders, M.J., Groenendaal, F. & De Vries, L.S. (2009): Preterm arterial ischaemic stroke. *Semin. Fetal Neonatal Med.* **14**, 272–277.

Burns, C.M., Rutherford, M.A., Boardman, J.P. & Cowan, F.M. (2008): Patterns of cerebral injury and neurodevelopmental outcomes after symptomatic neonatal hypoglycemia. *Pediatrics* **122**, 65–74.

Counsell, S.J., Edwards, A.D., Chew, A.T., *et al.* (2008): Specific relations between neurodevelopmental abilities and white matter microstructure in children born preterm. *Brain* **131**, 3201–3208.

Fransson, P., Skiöld, B., Horsch, S., *et al.* (2007): Resting-state networks in the infant brain. *Proc. Natl. Acad. Sci. USA* **104**, 15531–15536.

Govaert, P., Ramenghi, L., Taal, R., *et al.* (2009): Diagnosis of perinatal stroke. I: Definitions, differential diagnosis and registration. *Acta Paediatr.* **98**, 1556–1567.

Groenendaal, F., Veenhoven, R.H., van der Grond, J., *et al.* (1994): Cerebral lactate and N-acetyl-aspartate/choline ratios in asphyxiated full-term neonates demonstrated in vivo using proton magnetic resonance spectroscopy. *Pediatr. Res.* **35**, 148–151.

Ramenghi, L.A. & Hüppi, P.S. (2009): Imaging of the neonatal brain. In: *Foetal and Neonatal Neurology and Neurosurgery*, eds. M.I. Levene & F.A. Chevernak, pp. 68–103. London–Edinburgh: Churchill Livingstone.

Ramenghi, L.A., Fumagalli, M., Righini, A., *et al.* (2007): Magnetic resonance imaging assessment of brain maturation in preterm neonates with punctate white matter lesions. *Neuroradiology* **49**, 161–167.

Ramenghi, L.A., Mosca, F., Counsell, S. & Rutherford, M. (2005): Magnetic resonance imaging of the brain in preterm infants. In: *Pediatric Neuroradiology*, ed. Paolo Tortori Donati, pp. 199–234. Berlin: Springer.

Rutherford, M. (2001): *MRI of the Neonatal Brain*. London: Saunders.

Rutherford, M.A., Pennock, J.M., Counsell, S.J., *et al.* (1998): Abnormal magnetic resonance signal in the internal capsule predicts poor neurodevelopmental outcome in infants with hypoxic-ischaemic encephalopathy. *Pediatrics* **102**, 323–328.

Rutherford, M., Ramenghi, L.A., Edwards, A.D., *et al.* (2010a): Assessment of brain tissue injury after moderate hypothermia in neonates with hypoxic-ischaemic encephalopathy: a nested substudy of a randomised controlled trial. *Lancet Neurol.* **9,** 39–45.

Rutherford, M.A., Supramaniam, V., Ederise, A., *et al.* (2010b): Magnetic resonance imaging of white matter diseases of prematurity. *Neuroradiology* **52,** 505–521.

## Chapter 4

# Diffusion MR techniques to study the neonatal brain

Nora Tusor, Serena Counsell and Mary Rutherford

*Imaging Sciences Department, MRC Clinical Sciences Centre, Imperial College London, London, UK*
m.rutherford@imperial.ac.uk

### Summary

This article makes the following key points: (*i*) Diffusion tensor imaging (DTI) is easy to perform on the neonatal brain and should be part of the routine magnetic resonance (MR) examination. (*ii*) Apparent diffusion coefficient (ADC) values decrease and fractional anisotropy (FA) values increase with increasing age, reflecting brain maturation. (*iii*) Diffusion-weighted imaging (DWI) is clinically useful for identifying ischaemic tissue in the neonatal brain, the pattern of which can predict outcome. (*iv*) ADC values should always be measured along with visual analysis of the DW images. (*v*) ADC values $< 1.0 \times 10^{-3}/mm^2/s$ are associated with hemispheric white matter (WM) infarction and values $< 0.8 \times 10^{-3}/mm^2/s$ with thalamic damage. (*vi*) Techniques such as DTI, 3T imaging, and high-b-value imaging have important applications for clinical neonatology.

### Introduction

MR imaging (MRI) of the neonatal brain is a relatively new field, but many publications now illustrate its role in defining malformations, establishing patterns of perinatal injury, and predicting outcome (Barkovich, 1992; Kuenzle *et al.*, 1994; Mercuri *et al.*, 2000; Rutherford *et al.*, 1996, 1998).

MRI provides detailed information about the pattern of lesions following perinatal brain injury (Barkovich, 1992; Kuenzle *et al.*, 1994; Rutherford *et al.*, 1996; Rutherford, 2002) and is an excellent predictor of outcome in infants with hypoxic-ischaemic encephalopathy (HIE) (Rutherford *et al.*, 1998; Mercuri *et al.*, 1999, 2000; Boichot *et al.*, 2006; Liauw *et al.*, 2008). Conventional MRI has also been used to study perinatal stroke (Fig. 1). Hemiplegia develops later if there is involvement of three sites: hemispheric WM, basal ganglia and thalami (BGT), and posterior limb of the internal capsule (PLIC) (Mercuri *et al.*, 1999; Rutherford, 2002). In preterm infants with unilateral focal lesions the development of hemiplegia is related to the MR signal intensity within the ipsilateral PLIC at term-equivalent age (De Vries *et al.*, 1999). DWI may also help in predicting outcome by detecting abnormal signal intensities in the corticospinal tracts that precede the development of Wallerian degeneration (De Vries *et al.*, 2005).

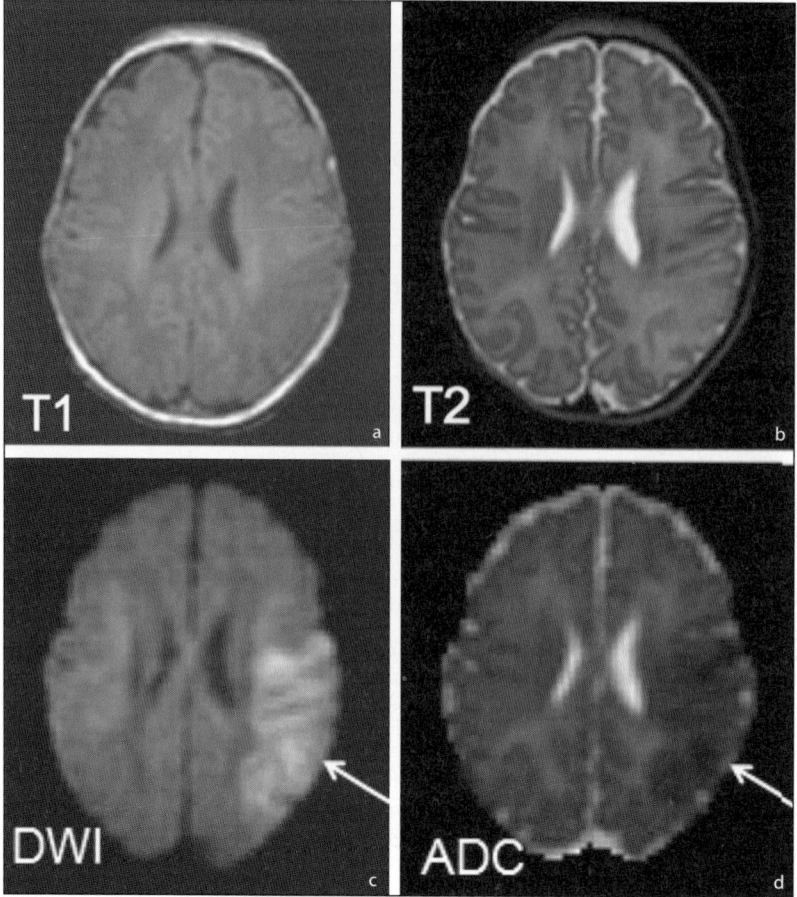

*Fig. 1. Left middle cerebral artery infarction in a 5-day-old infant. The abnormalities are subtle on the T1-weighted (SE 15/500) (a) and T2-weighted (FSE 4200/210) (b) images, but obvious on the DWI (c) and ADC map (d).*

## Practical issues

Successful imaging of the neonatal brain requires careful preparation of the infant and knowledge of the normally developing brain (Rutherford, 2002). These issues are not insurmountable, but require close cooperation between radiologist, radiographer, and neonatologist.

Neonates are not able to cooperate, yet a successful image relies on a still baby. To this end neonates may be successfully imaged during natural sleep, following a feed, or more successfully under light sedation with, for instance, chloral hydrate. All the neonates, sedated or not, should be monitored during scanning with MR-compatible pulse oximetry and electrocardiogram (ECG). A qualified paediatrician should be in attendance throughout the scan.

Excessive noise, particularly with fast sequences, may wake a sleeping infant or even harm the developing auditory system and ear protection should be used. We use mouldable dental putty as individualized earplugs and neonatal earmuffs (Natus MiniMuffs, <www.natus.com>). Infants may move even when asleep: moulded air bags or foam placed snugly around the infant's head will keep this to a minimum. Swaddling the infants will keep them warm and also reduce movements.

All the usual metal checks need to be carried out with particular attention, in this population, to the presence of intravenous lines, long lines, electroencephalogram (EEG) scalp electrodes, intraventricular shunts, and metal fasteners on baby clothes.

Neonates are small, the average term-born neonate weighs approximately 3.5 kg. Improved signal to noise will be obtained by using as small a coil as possible. In the absence of a dedicated paediatric coil, an adult knee coil is well suited; however these may not be large enough to accommodate an endotracheal tube in infants who are ventilated.

MR sequences will need to be adjusted for neonatal brain imaging. The neonatal brain has high water content, and tissue signal intensity contrasts are very different from those of the mature adult brain. The neonatal brain is largely unmyelinated, but reaches near-adult levels of myelination by the end of the second year. The pathologies of the immature brain also differ. Abnormalities are often symmetrical and may be mistaken for normal appearances by the inexperienced observer. In addition, the evolution of perinatal pathology takes place in a background of a brain that is developing rapidly both in terms of actual size and in its tissue properties.

## What is diffusion?

Diffusion MRI is a method that produces *in vivo* images weighted with the local microstructural characteristics of water diffusion.

The random, translational motion of water molecules, because of their thermal energy (Brownian motion) in a homogenous medium (such as cerebrospinal fluid), is equal in all directions and is termed isotropic diffusion. Meanwhile the diffusion of water molecules in tissue with an ordered microstructure (such as WM) is direction-dependent and anisotropic (Fig. 2) (Moseley *et al.*, 1990).

In a free fluid, individual molecules travel randomly over a distance that can be described statistically by the diffusion coefficient. The diffusion coefficient depends on the temperature, the mass of the molecules, and the viscosity of the medium. During typical diffusion times of 50–100 ms, water molecules in brain tissue move over distances of around 1–15 µm, bouncing, crossing, and interacting with many tissue components, such as cell membranes, fibres, and macromolecules. These processes impede motion so that, in tissue, the distance travelled by a water molecule due to diffusion is less than that in free water (at the same temperature). Hence,

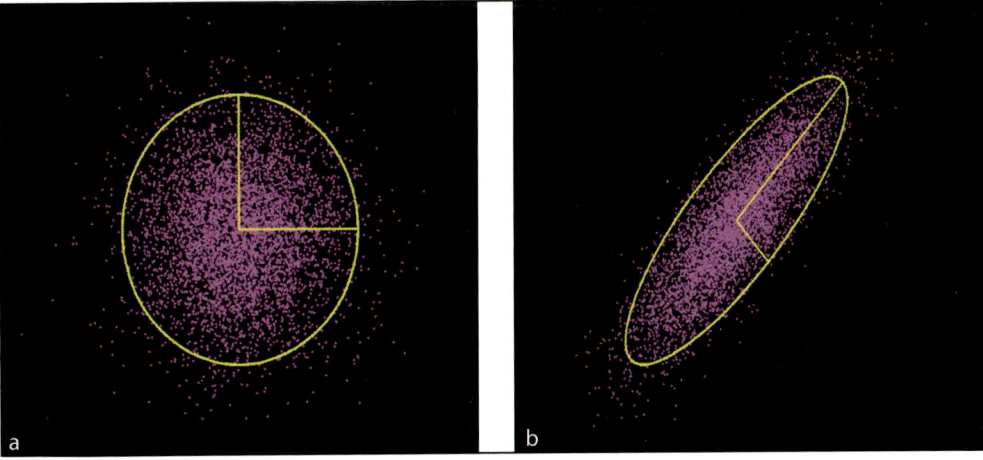

*Fig. 2. Isotropic (**a**) and anisotropic (**b**) diffusion (<www.fmrib.ox.ac.uk>).*

the diffusion of water molecules *in vivo* provides information regarding structural features and tissue organization. As the diffusion coefficient obtained in tissue depends on the local microstructural environment and on the choice of diffusion weighting, it is termed the ADC.

In the presence of a spatially varying magnetic field, random motion of protons in diffusing water molecules results in dephasing of the MR signal, producing a reduction in its amplitude. Since spatially varying magnetic fields are used for slice selection and spatial encoding in all MR images, diffusion of water molecules results in a reduction in signal intensity in all images, although the effect is normally quite small. By deliberately applying large magnetic field gradients in particular directions diffusion can be made the dominant image contrast mechanism, and provide visualization of variations in diffusion, including their directional dependence.

In order to examine anisotropy, a minimum of 6 non-collinear directions of diffusion sensitization are obtained, which is DTI. A mathematical tensor can be calculated that describes the motion of water in the studied tissue (Besser *et al.*, 1994). This tensor can be conceptualized as an ellipsoid, of which the long axis represents the direction with the highest diffusivity; the magnitude of its diffusivity is given by the major eigenvalue ($\lambda 1$) and its direction is called the major eigenvector. The diffusivity along the major axis is called axial diffusivity. Perpendiculars to the major eigenvector are the two short axes: the median and minimum eigenvectors, with their eigenvalues ($\lambda 2$, $\lambda 3$) (LeBihan *et al.*, 2001; Mori *et al.*, 2006). Diffusivities along the minor axes are often averaged to produce a measure of radial diffusivity. Using DTI, the separate values of $\lambda 1$, $\lambda 2$, $\lambda 3$ in an imaging voxel can be quantified. Averaged mean diffusivity (Dav) then can be calculated as one-third of the trace of the diffusion tensor, ($\lambda 1$, $\lambda 2$, $\lambda 3$)/3 and provides the overall magnitude of water diffusion. Dav is a useful parameter that can serve as an indicator of brain maturation and/or injury (Hüppi *et al.*, 1998; McKinstry *et al.*, 2002).

The most commonly used measure of diffusion is anisotropy. Fractional anisotropy (FA) is the fraction of the magnitude of diffusion that can be attributed to anisotropic diffusion. FA values range between 0 and 1. An FA value close to zero represents diffusion that is equal in all directions; whereas a value close to 1 suggests diffusion that is highly directionally dependent, such as along a major WM fibre bundle. FA increases with WM maturation, but decreases with cortical maturation.

**The normal neonatal brain**

DWI techniques have been used to study the normal neonatal brain (Tanner *et al.*, 2000; Forbes *et al.*, 2002; Miller *et al.*, 2003; Boichot *et al.*, 2006; Bartha *et al.*, 2007). In neonates ADC values are higher than in more mature brain. There is regional variation: ADC values are lower in gray matter (GM) than in myelinated WM and the highest in unmyelinated WM. Representative ADC values for normal-term brain are shown in Table 1. All the above studies obtained DWI at 1.5T with two b-values (0 and 1,000 mm$^2$/s). In Forbes' study of 40 children from birth to 1 year, 14 infants were born at term, but all were scanned for clinical reasons and were therefore not true controls. Their ADC values for subcortical frontal WM were slightly higher than the values in Table 1 (median 1.88 compared to $1.6 \times 10^{-3}$/mm$^2$/s, respectively), but for the PLIC, ADC values were comparable (median 1.09 *vs.* $1.0 \times 10^{-3}$/mm$^2$/s). Forbes *et al.* also noted an increase in ADC values within anterior WM compared with posterior WM. The median ADC in controls was $1.6 \times 10^{-3}$/mm$^2$/s for anterior WM, which was not significantly different from the $1.55 \times 10^{-3}$/mm$^2$/s for posterior WM. Variation in regions of interest which were measured within the WM may explain some of the differences between these studies. Tanner's study measured ADC values in 10 term-born neurologically-normal neonates less than 43 days old, and their values for anterior WM were comparable to those in Table 1 (1.62 vs. 1.6–10⁻³/mm²/s). Bartha's study of 14 neonates with normal imaging using 6-direction DTI with b-values of 0 and 700 mm²/s showed a mean ADC value across the neonates of $1.19 \times 10^{-3}$/mm²/s for the basal ganglia and $0.98 \times 10^{-3}$/mm²/s for the thalami and $1.46 \times 10^{-3}$/mm²/s and $1.48 \times 10^{-3}$/mm²/s for the posterior and frontal white matter, respectively. All neonates had normal short-term outcome at 14 months of age, but were recruited after perinatal complications. Winter et al. (2007), as part of a study of neonates with HIE, studied 30 normal controls, neonates without neurologic signs, and obtained very similar ADC values.

ADC values reach mature adult levels by about 2 years, although small decreases may still be found until early adulthood.

There are few DTI studies of the normal-term brain. Anisotropy of WM tracts has been identified prior to myelination (Hüppi et al., 1998; Mukherjee et al., 2002; Miller et al., 2003; Bartha et al., 2007). Measurements of regional anisotropy (RA) are lower than in the adult brain in WM and in central grey matter (DeLano et al., 2002; Provenzale et al., 2007; Bartha et al., 2007).

Table 1. ADC values [median (range)] in different brain regions

| Region | Controls ADC ($\times 10^{-3}$/mm²/s) | All patients ADC ($\times 10^{-3}$/mm²/s) |
|---|---|---|
| Thalami | 1 (1–1.15) | 1 (0.5–1.4) |
| VLN | 0.88 (0.76–0.95) | 0.85 (0.39–1.2) |
| Lentiform | 1.1 (1–1.3) | 1.05 (0.5–1.65) |
| PLIC | 1 (0.83–1.2) | 0.9 (0.48–1.5) |
| WM CSO | 1.5 (1.3–1.7) | 1.43 (0.5–2.0) |
| WM (ant) | 1.6 (1.5–1.7) | 1.5 (0.6–1.95) |
| WM (post) | 1.55 (1.35–1.85) | 1.5 (0.5–1.9) |
| Cerebellar hemispheres | 1.1 (1–1.25) | 1 (0.8–1.3) |
| Vermis | 0.97 (0.8–1.2) | 0.98 (0.7–1.2) |
| Brainstem | 0.98 (0.86–1.1) | 0.92 (0.5–1.25) |

VLN: ventrolateral nuclei of thalami; CSO: centrum semi-ovale; ant: anterior; post: posterior.

## Clinical applications

### Focal infarction or stroke

The incidence of neonatal arterial ischaemic stroke is estimated to be in the range of 1 in 4,000 deliveries (Lynch et al., 2009). These neonates have typically normal Apgar scores, but present around day 2 of life with seizures that might be contralateral to the site of the infarction and are usually clonic in nature (Mercuri et al., 1999; Sreenan et al., 2000), but can be subtle as well. On conventional T2-weighted images, loss of grey-white matter distinction may escape detection because of small lesion size or poor quality of images due to motion artefacts.

DWI has been used to assess tissue injury in neonates with perinatal stroke (Cowan et al., 1994; Krishnamoorthy et al., 2000) as DW sequences have been shown to display intracellular oedema with high sensitivity, which is the initial finding in perinatal stroke (Fig. 3); also, echo planar images (EPI) can be acquired in few minutes and hence patient motion is less likely to create problems during these examinations.

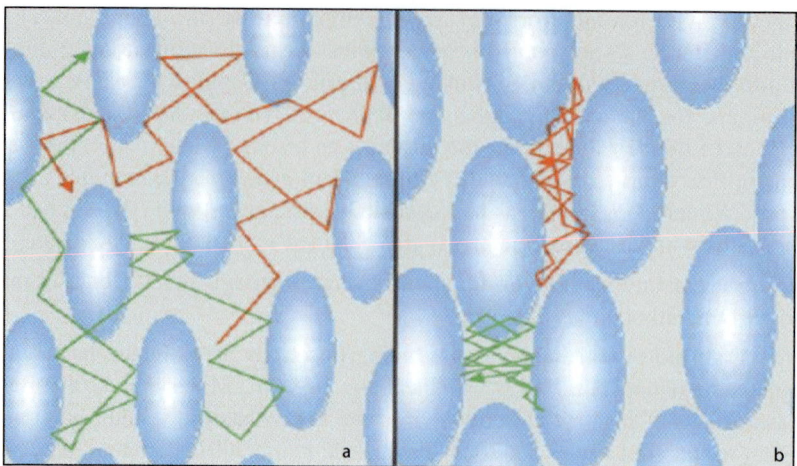

*Fig. 3. Normal diffusion (**a**) and reduction of diffusivity in the extracellular space following ischaemia due to cytotoxic oedema (**b**).*

DWI can detect acute ischaemic injury even before T2 signal changes are appreciated as an area of increased signal on DWI with low signal on ADC map. The ADC values may decrease to approximately 30–50 per cent of normal (Fig. 4). The evolution of diffusion abnormality in perinatal stroke is consistent with and similar to that seen in adults (Fiesbach *et al.*, 2002), although pseudonormalization has been reported to occur faster in neonates than in adults (around 5 days in neonates versus 2 weeks in mature adult brain), which may be due to the reduced amount of cell membranes within the unmyelinated newborn brain (Mader *et al.*, 2002). During pseudonormalization abnormal signal intensity gradually reduces by the end of the first week as the conventional imaging appearances become more abnormal.

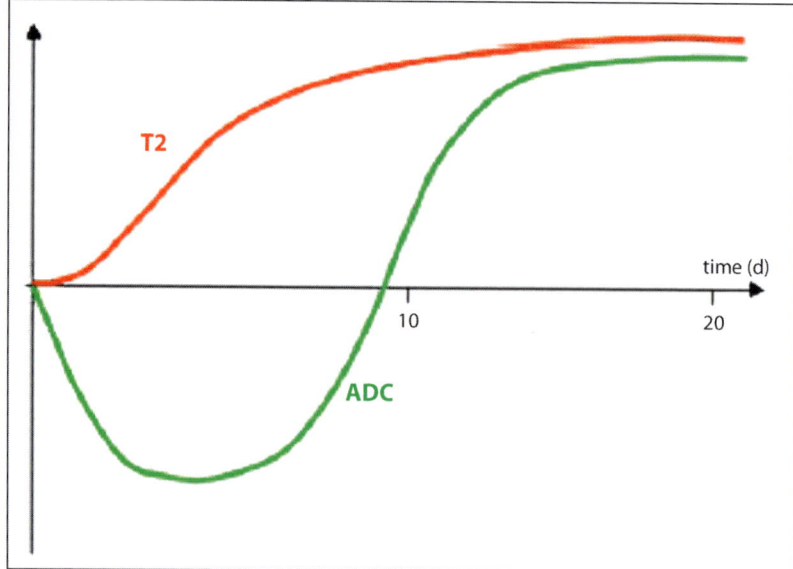

*Fig. 4. The time course of ADC and T2 change after arterial occlusion.*

In case of perinatal stroke it is difficult to time the onset of infarction as the aetiology is poorly understood and the seizures may not be clinically obvious until the neonate is 48 hours of age. Dudink *et al.* (2008) analyzed 43 scans from 21 term-born neonates with unilateral infarction and found that the pattern of changes on conventional and DWI are consistent among patients, suggesting that the onset of infarction in symptomatic term-born infants occurs within a limited time frame around birth.

DWI may appear to overestimate the size of a perinatal infarct, but this is difficult to prove in the face of a growing and developing brain. Registration of serially acquired images have shown excessive growth in and around areas of infarction after perinatal stroke (Rutherford *et al.*, 1997a, 1997b), but the infarcted hemisphere is always smaller and shows less myelin on follow-up images.

Mercuri *et al.* investigated the prognostic factors following neonatal cerebral infarction. The antenatal and perinatal risk factors, clinical course, EEG and MRI findings were studied in 24 children with evidence of cerebral infarction on neonatal conventional MRI. It was found that the extent of lesion on MRI, in particular the concomitant involvement of hemisphere, PLIC, and BG, was always associated with an abnormal outcome, whereas the involvement of only one or two of the three tended to be associated with a normal outcome (Mercuri *et al.*, 1999).

Kirton *et al.* studied the role of restricted diffusion in the corticospinal tracts in predicting outcome in 14 neonates with acute perinatal arterial stroke with > 12 months' outcome. It was found that poor outcome correlated with decreased ADC values in ipsilesional descending corticospinal tract (Kirton *et al.*, 2007). The finding of association between chronic Wallerian degeneration and hemiparesis was confirmed by other studies (De Vries *et al.*, 2005) (Fig. 5).

**Hypoxic-ischaemic insult**

After a perinatal hypoxic-ischaemic insult, abnormalities detected with conventional MRI may take several days to evolve, a period during which maximum benefit from neuroprotective strategies, such as hypothermia, to modify brain injury may be obtained and when important clinical decisions have to be made. Very early confirmation of the site and severity of tissue injury enables appropriate targeting of therapeutic interventions in a far more specific way than is currently available. In addition, even established abnormalities may not be obvious to the inexperienced radiologist. An additional and more objective method of assessing tissue integrity early after injury, such as DWI, is therefore very useful.

In infants with a global hypoxic-ischaemic insult, the most frequent site of injury is to the central grey matter (GM). Bilateral BGT lesions are strongly associated with the development of motor impairment and the extent of the lesions is closely related to the severity of that impairment (Rutherford *et al.*, 1996). Even moderate BGT lesions are usually associated with significant motor impairment in the form of quadriplegic cerebral palsy (Fig. 6). Moderate WM abnormalities are associated with relatively good outcome, normal motor development, but higher risk of cognitive impairment. However, severe WM infarction leads to cognitive impairment, but less-severe motor impairment (Fig. 7) (Mercuri *et al.*, 2000; Cowan *et al.*, 2003).

It is therefore very important to be able to correctly diagnose the presence of BGT or WM lesions after an asphyxial event. It is essential to consider the timing of the injury, the age of the infant, the conventional image's appearances, and to look at the DWI in addition to measuring the ADC to maximize the predictive abilities of diffusion techniques to correctly identify ischaemic tissue.

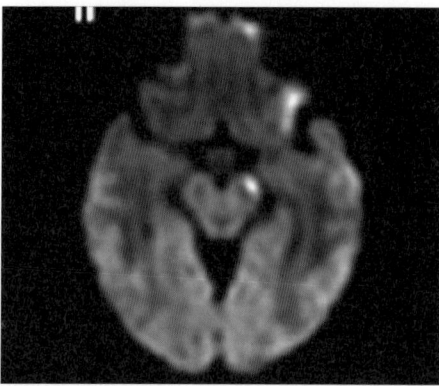

*Fig. 5. Abnormal signal intensity in the cerebral peduncles is a strong predictor of subsequent development of Wallerian degeneration and hemiplegia in case of perinatal stroke.*

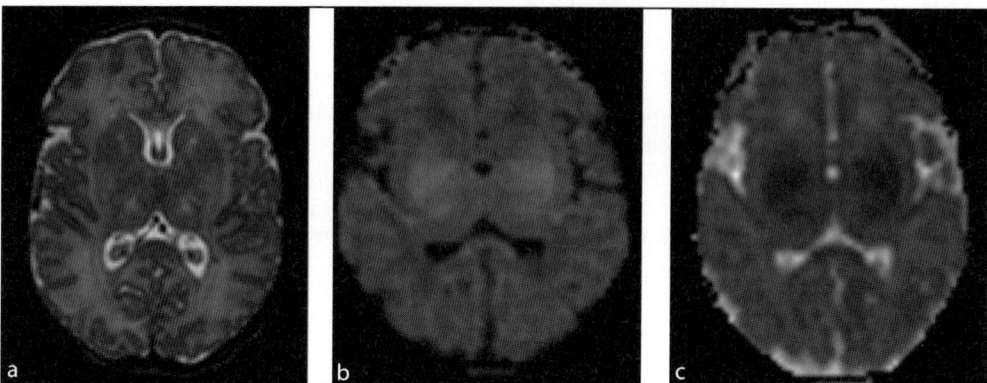

*Fig. 6. Abnormal BGT on T2-weighted (a), DWI (b), and ADC map (c). BGT lesion in HIE is associated with abnormal motor development.*

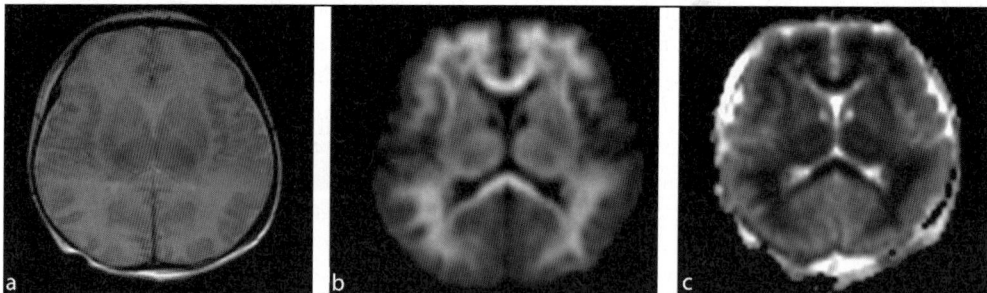

*Fig. 7. WM injury on conventional (a), DWI (b), and ADC (c) imaged on day 2 after history of decreased foetal movements. WM lesion in HIE is associated with higher risk of cognitive impairment.*

There are relatively few studies using DWI in infants with HIE and these have had conflicting results (Forbes *et al.*, 2000; Barkovich *et al.*, 2001; Wolf *et al.*, 2001; McKinstry *et al.*, 2002; Takeoka *et al.*, 2002; Zarifi *et al.*, 2002; Vermeulen *et al.*, 2008). DWI may show obvious visual abnormalities following bilateral WM infarction in HIE, but not if the BGT are also affected. In these infants a clue may be found by observing the appearance of the normal cerebellum (Vermeulen *et al.*, 2003) and measuring the ADC values will correctly detect the presence of ischaemic tissue. DWI appearances in the presence of isolated but clinically significant BGT lesions are less consistent. Abnormal areas may shift during the first two weeks after injury (Barkovich et al., 2006). Any abnormality within the BGT on an individual ADC map is likely to underestimate the eventual lesion load within the BGT seen on later conventional imaging (Fig. 8).

The evolution of ADC values in hypoxic-ischaemic brain lesions was demonstrated by McKinstry and colleagues, who determined the average ADC over all brain lesions at three time-points within the first 11 postnatal days in ten neonates with neonatal encephalopathy. The ADC values decreased to a minimum at approximately 2–3 days of postnatal age and then increased, reaching normal values (pseudonormalization) on approximately the seventh postnatal day (McKinstry et al., 2002). Rutherford et al. (2004) studied the relationship between contemporaneous DWI and conventional MRI in 63 term-born neonates with HIE and compared the results to control term-born infants. DWI was acquired using single-shot EPI at multiple levels. Fifteen slices of 5-mm thickness were obtained (repetition time [TR] 6,000 ms, echo time [TE] 110 ms, field of view (FOV) 24 cm, b-values of 0 and 1,000 s/mm$^2$) in three orthogonal directions. In infants with HIE, ADC values were significantly reduced in the first week after severe injury to either WM ($P < 0.0001$) or BGT ($P < 0.0001$), but values normalized at the end of the first week and then increased during week two. Winter et al. (2007) studied the ADC pseudonormalization time in 12 neonates with poor outcome following HIE and in 30 term-born control subjects. The pseudonormalization time in their cohort ranged between 8 and 10 postnatal days. Although abnormally decreased ADC values may be present from approximately 2 days to almost 1 week of postnatal age, abnormally elevated values may not be apparent until late in the second week of life.

It is well-known that abnormal signal intensity in the PLIC on conventional MRI predicts poor motor outcome in term infants after perinatal asphyxia (Fig. 9) (Rutherford et al., 1998). To establish the supplemental role of DWI in predicting outcome in neonatal encephalopathy Vermeulen et al. (2008) measured the ADC value in 14 brain regions between days 1 and 45 in 46 infants with neonatal HIE and also assessed the motor outcome at the age of 2 years. They found that infants with poor outcome had significantly lower ADC values ($< 0.8 \times 10^{-3}/\text{mm}^2/\text{s}$) in the PLIC during the first week of life (Fig. 10).

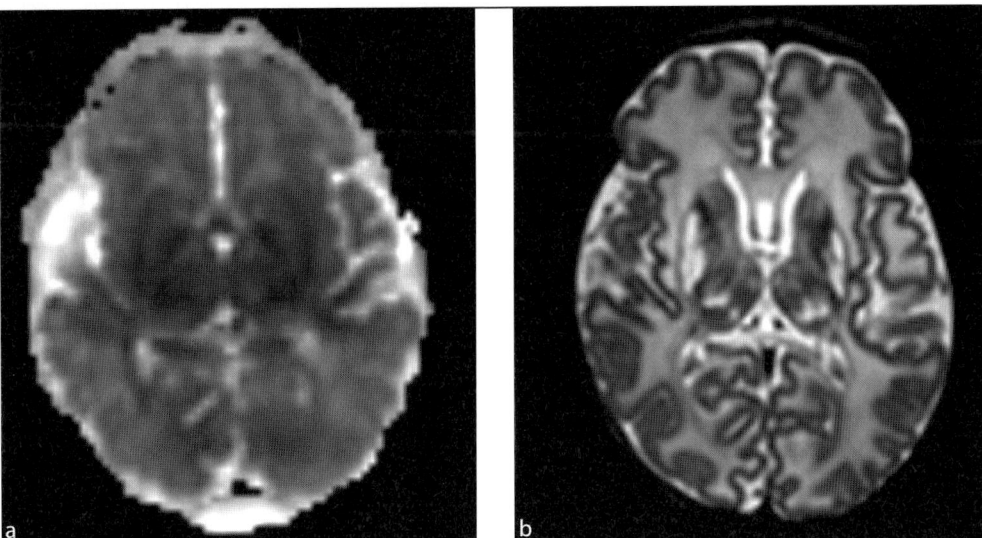

Fig. 8. Early DTI on day 3 (**a**) underestimates the BGT lesion appearing by day 22 on T2-weighted image (**b**).

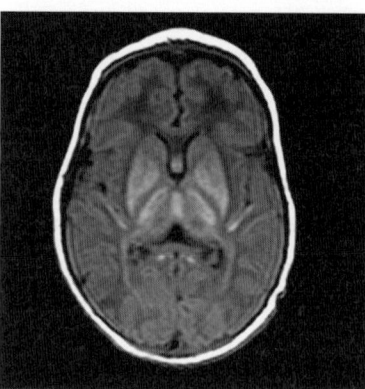

*Fig. 9. Abnormal signal intensity in the PLIC predicts abnormal motor outcome in infants with HIE. Sensitivity = 0.9; specificity = 1.0.*

DTI may improve the ability to detect abnormal tissue by another parameter: the FA. Anisotropy increases with age as radial diffusivity perpendicular to the tracts decreases within the tissue. ADC and FA values were studied by Ward and colleagues in 20 infants with HIE and 7 normal-term controls. The scans were performed during the first 3 weeks of life. It was found that during the first week FA values were decreased in both severe and moderate WM and BGT injury, whereas ADC values were reduced only in severe WM injury and some severe BGT injury. Meanwhile ADC values pseudonormalized by the second week of life, FA values continued to decrease (Ward *et al.*, 2006). This suggests that a combination of ADC and FA values derived from DTI combined with visual analysis of conventional imaging offers the best approach for identifying and timing all abnormal tissue. However, it is unlikely that this approach could serve as a useful basis for identifying infants for potential early interventions such as hypothermia, given that current protocols are starting therapeutic hypothermia within 6 hours after delivery, with passive cooling starting prior to this when possible. It is unrealistic at present to expect infants to have safely undergone a good-quality MR scan within this time. However, it may provide a useful method for monitoring the effects of treatment both during and after intervention.

Potential therapies at present concentrate on acute intervention, but there is evidence to suggest ongoing injury in the neonate with HIE that may be amenable to later treatments. In a study of infants who sustained BGT lesions perinatally, it was found that white matter appearances, which were initially normal with normal ADC, deteriorated during the second week. ADC values, instead of decreasing within the white matter as would normally happen with increasing postnatal age, actually *increased* (Rutherford *et al.*, 2005). This phenomenon can be witnessed when looking at serially-obtained conventional images when initially normally-appearing white matter eventually atrophies in the presence of severe basal ganglia lesions. These late changes are consistent with delayed injury occurring as a consequence of an initial insult to the BGT. This suggests that there may still be scope for intervening during the first few days after perinatal hypoxic-ischaemic insult. These interventions may have to be targeted towards white matter and possibly to different mechanisms of cell death (*e.g.*, apoptosis and necrosis).

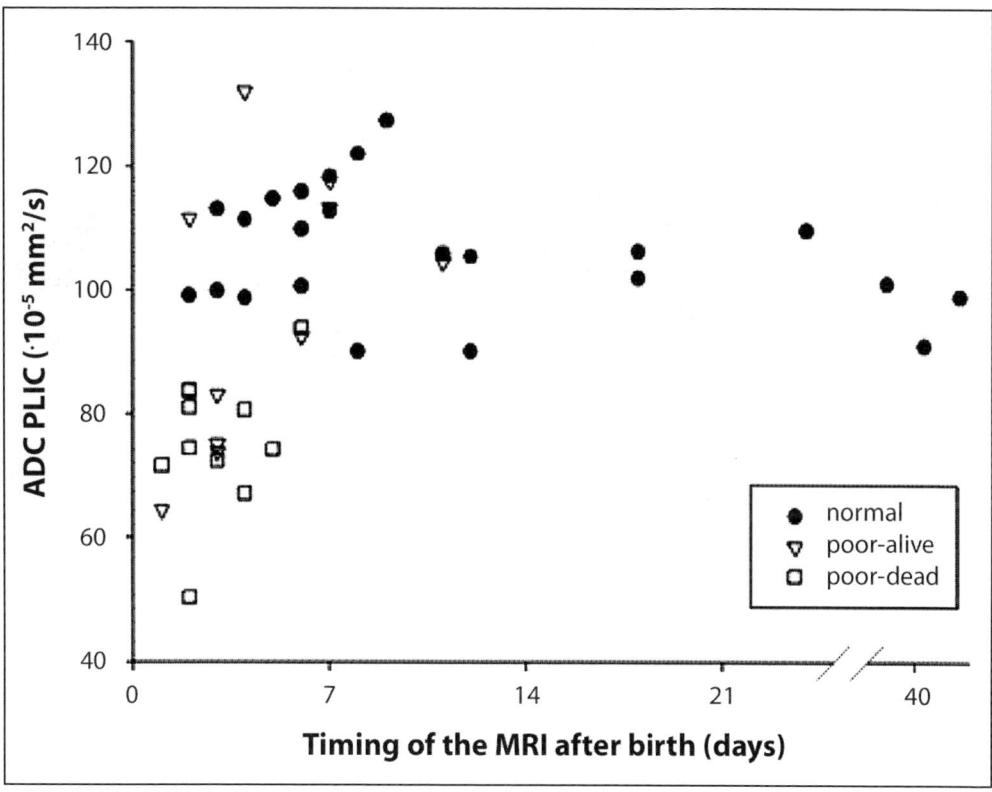

*Fig. 10. ADC values predict outcome in HIE (Vermeulen et al., 2008).*

**Congenital malformations**

In addition to identifying areas of acute ischaemia in the immature brain, DTI has some additional clinical roles. In infants with callosal agenesis, DTI may be used to identify abnormal tracts, which run medial to the lateral ventricles, giving them their characteristic shape, the so-called Probst bundles. In infants with Joubert's syndrome, brainstem DTI has been used to demonstrate the absence of decussation of the pyramidal tracts and abnormal orientation of superior cerebellar peduncles (Poretti et al., 2007) In congenital central hypoventilation syndrome DTI studies have revealed abnormal FA at multiple sites within the cerebellum and brainstem (Kumar et al., 2008).

**Metabolic disorders**

Conventional MRI is able to identify brain malformations that may accompany some metabolic disorders, such as callosal agenesis in non-ketotic hyperglycinaemia (NKH) or cortical migration defects in peroxisomal disorders such as Zellweger syndrome. WM in these infants may have a long T1 and long T2, which may be reflected in increased ADC values. Occasionally the results of DWI are more enlightening and show more distinct abnormalities. These may be reversible with treatment and could potentially be used to monitor therapy. A combination of vasogenic and cytotoxic oedema has been reported in an infant with Menke disease, an inherited disorder of copper metabolism (Barnerias et al., 2008).

In infants with maple-syrup urine disease (MSUD), DWI is pathognomonic, resulting in a 'map' of actively myelinating areas (Fig. 11) (Cavalleri et al., 2002). There are also reports of abnormal DWI in NKH (Khong et al., 2003; Shah et al., 2005) This is an important finding as the areas of abnormality (*e.g.*, cerebral peduncles, internal capsule) may mimic those found with more straightforward HIE, and the diagnosis of NKH may be missed. This further emphasizes the need to fully investigate any infant presenting with neonatal seizures, not only by means of a careful history and examination, but also by metabolic investigation as well as neuroimaging, which should, where possible, be MR imaging and include DWI.

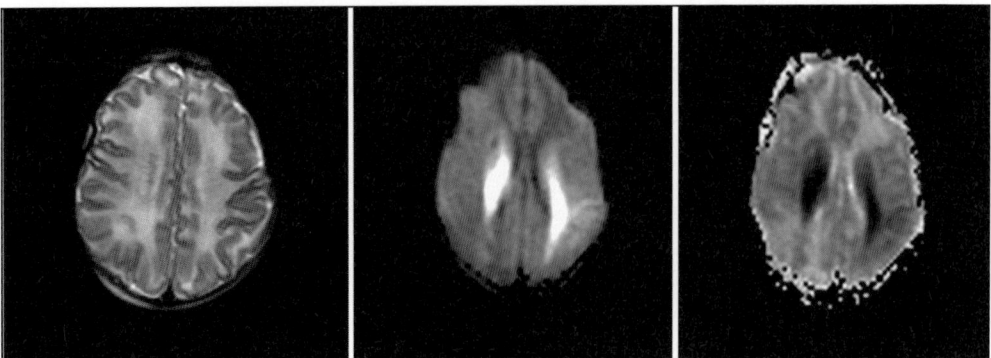

*Fig. 11. Abnormal signal intensity in the myelinating tracts in maple-syrup disease.*

**Preterm brain development**

Data from studies from the USA, Europe, and Australia have all revealed poorer educational outcome in preterm children than in term controls (Ment *et al.*, 2009). At school entry, minor developmental impairment has been diagnosed in 30–40 per cent of preterm children and major disabilities in almost 20 per cent of preterm children (Allen *et al.*, 2008; Larroque *et al.*, 2008; Saigal *et al.*, 2008; Neubauer *et al.*, 2008; Voss *et al.*, 2007). Injury is common in the preterm brain. The most common focal injuries in the preterm population are cystic periventricular leucomalacia (PVL) and germinal matrix/intraventricular haemorrhage. More-diffuse injury in the periventricular WM occurs in up to 50 per cent of very-low-birth-weight infants (Ment *et al.*, 2009). There are relatively few MR studies in preterm brain pathology because of difficulties in safely transporting and scanning small and often sick preterm neonates.

Hüppi *et al.* have compared 20 preterm infants born between 27–31 weeks, 10 with normal brain appearances and 10 with evidence of WM injury and found regional reductions in anisotropy in the WM group. Differences in ADC in preterm infants with DEHSI at term-equivalent age have been found (Counsell *et al.*, 2006), and Krishnan and colleagues reported significant negative correlation between ADC values in the centrum semiovale and the Griffiths Mental Developmental Scales score at the age of 2 years (Krishnan *et al.*, 2007). These findings were confirmed by Counsell *et al.* (2008) using TBSS.

In a study with region-of-interest analysis using DTI, Dudink *et al.* (2007) have shown that FA values in the WM of preterm infants increase with increasing gestational age. DTI studies of the very immature brain have shown increased relative anisotropy (RA) in the developing cortex consistent with the simple radiating organization of fibres (McKinstry *et al.*, 2002). Gimenez *et al.* (2008) noted higher FA values in the preterm group at term-equivalent age in areas corresponding to fibre tracts of the neurosensory pathways, such as the inferior frontal occipital fascicle, stria terminalis, fornix, optic radiations, inferior longitudinal fascicle, and lateral geniculate nucleus, suggesting that these areas mature more rapidly in preterm infants on account of increased early experience.

In preterm infants with overt WM pathology such as PVL, DWI has been used to identify areas of restricted diffusion in WM prior to cyst formation (Inder *et al.*, 1999; Roelants-van Rijn *et al.*, 2001) when ultrasound or conventional MRI showed no or nonspecific abnormalities (Fig. 12). Histologic changes in the acute phase of PVL alter WM microstructure and water diffusivity, and a reduced ADC in the periventricular WM in an otherwise normal preterm brain is considered an early indicator of WM injury (Hüppi & Dubois, 2006). DWI may also show areas of restricted diffusion adjacent to established cystic lesions in PVL and has also been used to identify abnormal WM in areas distant from cystic lesions, the ADC values in these areas being higher than in normal tissue (Counsell *et al.*, 2003). Anisotropy of the WM also changes after both focal and diffuse WM injury. In the chronic stage of PVL, decreased relative anisotropy may be detected and FA maps may show disruption of WM tracts distant from the focal lesions detected on conventional imaging (Hüppi *et al.*, 2001). Arzoumanian and colleagues analyzed DTI values acquired at term-equivalent age and follow-up data at corrected age of 18–24 months on 137 preterm neonates and showed that FA values in the PLIC were significantly lower for preterm infants with cerebral palsy compared with those without cerebral palsy (Arzoumanian *et al.*, 2003).

## Advanced tools

### TBSS

Tract-based spatial statistics (TBSS) (Smith *et al.*, 2006) is an automated, observer-independent method for assessing FA in major WM tracts. After pre-processing steps (eddy current correction, brain extraction, fitting the tensor model, and calculating FA images), a common registration target is identified and all subjects' FA images are aligned to this target using nonlinear registration. The mean of all aligned FA images is then generated, creating the mean FA map. The standard adult protocol needs to be modified slightly for assessment of the neonatal brain, as it was found that registering the native FA data again to this mean FA map improves accuracy (Ball *et al.*, 2010). Importantly, standard adult templates are not useful in neonates, and so the mean FA map from the subject's dataset should always be used. The skeletonized mean FA is created by thinning the mean FA image. The mean FA skeleton that represents the centres of all tracts common to the group (Fig. 13 is 'thresholded' to a mean FA value of 0.15 in neonates (*vs.* 0.2 in adults) to include the major white matter pathways but exclude peripheral tracts, where there may be significant intersubject variability and/or partial volume effects with grey matter. Each subject's aligned FA image is projected onto the skeleton. Then multivariate voxel-wise statistics across subjects can be carried out on the voxels within the skeleton.

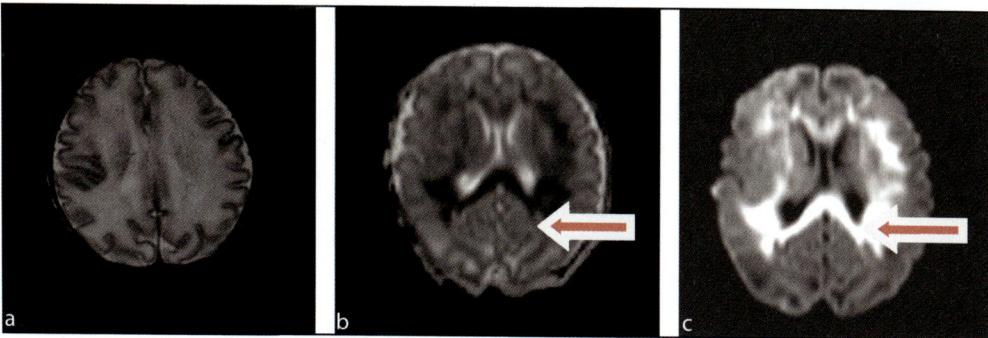

Fig. 12. PVL on day 6 on conventional MRI (*a*), DTI (*b*), and DWI (*c*).

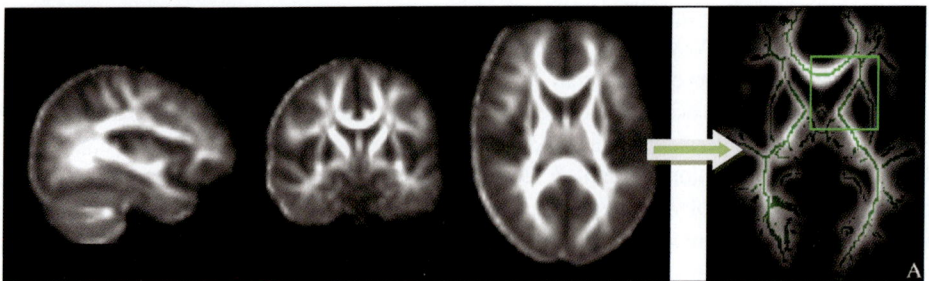

*Fig. 13. In TBSS following alignment the mean of all FA is generated and then thinned to create the skeletonized mean FA, which represents all the tracts common to the group (Smith et al., 2006).*

Recently, voxel-based approaches have been used to assess white matter in the preterm brain. Anjari and colleagues used TBSS in a cohort of 26 preterm infants without focal lesions imaged at term-equivalent age and found a number of regions in the preterm brain where anisotropy was lower compared to that of six infants born at term, including the frontal WM, centrum semiovale, posterior limb of the internal capsule, and the corpus callosum (Fig. 14) (Anjari *et al.*, 2007). This work suggests that widespread WM abnormalities are present in the brain of preterm infants, even in the absence of major focal lesions. To investigate the observed reduction in FA, the three eigenvectors of the diffusion tensor were also analysed. The regions that exhibited decreased FA showed elevated intermediate ($\lambda2$) and/or minor ($\lambda3$) eigenvalues, findings that are consistent with previous ROI analysis of DTI data from preterm and term-born control infants (Counsell *et al.*, 2006).

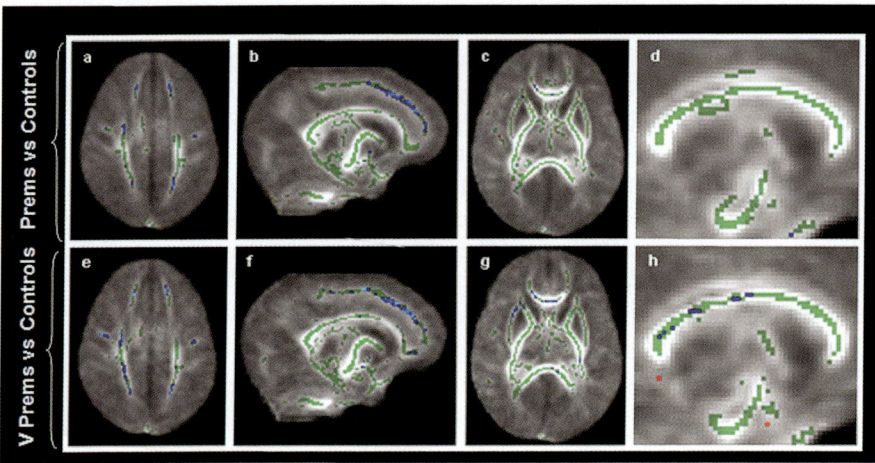

*Fig. 14. FA difference in preterm vs. term infants. Blue: FA significantly lower in the preterm group. Green: no difference in FA between groups (Anjari et al., 2007).*

Anjari *et al.* (2009) also used TBSS to investigate the association of acute and chronic lung disease (CLD) with WM abnormalities in preterm infants. By means of regression analysis to allow for the effects of gestational age (GA) and postmenstrual age (PMA), infants who suffered acute lung disease, defined as need for ventilation for $\geq 2$ days ($n = 10$), displayed a localized region of reduced FA within the genu of the corpus callosum, whereas infants with CLD, defined by the need for supplemental inspired oxygen at 36 weeks' postmenstrual age, showed reduced FA in the left inferior longitudinal fasciculus. These results showed that acute and chronic lung diseases are associated with specific abnormalities in the WM, suggesting that respiratory disease and its treatment may be a significant cause of subtle cerebral injury in preterm infants.

Ball *et al.* used TBSS with the modified registration method described above to further investigate the association between WM microstructural development and respiratory morbidity in preterm neonates scanned at term-equivalent age. They showed that CLD was associated with increased radial diffusivity (RD) and decreased FA and also that the global pattern of altered AD, RD, and FA was linearly associated with the length of respiratory support needed, even in the absence of CLD. By means of regression analysis to allow for the strong effects of increasing prematurity at birth, PMA at imaging, and altered WM microstructure at term-equivalent age, a more widespread association of CLD on both FA and RD was demonstrated, incorporating not only the inferior longitudinal fasciculus bilaterally, but also the corpus callosum and the centrum semiovale (Ball *et al.*, 2010).

Using TBSS, Counsell and colleagues investigated the neurodevelopmental abilities of 2-year-old children who were born preterm, showing that FA values in the isthmus and the body of the corpus callosum were significantly correlated with the overall DQ scores, values in the corpus callosum and right cingulum with the performance sub-scores, and values in the cingulum bilaterally, the fornix, the anterior commissure, the corpus callosum and the right uncinate fasciculus with the eye–hand coordination sub-scores. Reduction in FA may reflect reductions in myelination, axonal damage, or decreased fibre coherence (Counsell *et al.*, 2008).

TBSS may also be a powerful tool to assess the differences between treatment groups. Porter *et al.* (2010) used TBSS to assess the neuroprotective effect of cooling in a small cohort of 8 control infants, 10 cooled infants with HIE, and 10 non-cooled infants with HIE. When compared to controls, non-cooled infants had significantly reduced FA in many WM tracts throughout the brain: bilaterally in the anterior and posterior limb of the internal capsule; throughout the external capsule; the body of the corpus callosum; the cingulum; the fornix; the superior longitudinal fasciculus and the superior corona radiate; and the inferior longitudinal fasciculus on the left side. Meanwhile, when the cooled group of infants was compared to the control group, FA was significantly reduced only in the internal capsule. Comparing 10 cooled to 10 non-cooled infants with HIE, the investigators demonstrated that the non-cooled infants have significantly lower FA in several WM tracts, including the superior corona radiate, corpus callosum, internal capsule, external capsule, and optic radiations (Porter *et al.*, 2010). These data confirm that TBSS analysis of FA is a powerful tool to assess and compare WM tissue integrity between patient groups and they suggest that it is a suitable biomarker for early-phase trials of novel neuroprotective strategies.

**Tractography**

WM pathways in the brain exist in three dimensions, hence even sophisticated 2D representations, such as directionally encoded colour anisotropy maps, are intrinsically limited. Moreover these anisotropy maps cannot differentiate adjacent WM tracts that have the same fibre orientation. DTI tractography provides a potentially valuable tool to assess connectivity *in vivo*. By studying the preferred direction of water diffusion it is possible to infer the orientation of major WM fibre bundles.

Fibre tracking algorithms can be broadly classified into two types: *deterministic* and *probabilistic*.

In deterministic tractography the main assumption is that the direction of the eigenvector associated with the largest eigenvalue is aligned with the direction of the underlying fibre bundle. This algorithm proceeds from an initially determined point in the direction of the principal eigenvector from voxel to voxel. In deterministic tractography two sets of thresholds are often applied. The first is a minimum value of anisotropy: tracing is determined if the tract enters a region below this value. A second threshold is an angular threshold: the maximum angle a path can turn between each step to prevent impossible turns in fibre orientation (Jones et al., 2008). There are limitations to the deterministic approach, such as only one reconstructed trajectory per seed is produced and it may not show the branching of the WM tracts; voxels containing multiple fibres of different orientations have reduced net anisotropy; and fibre tracking can terminate the tractography, giving no indication of the confidence that one can assign to a reconstructed trajectory (Dudink et al., 2008).

In probabilistic tractography, instead of reconstructing a single trajectory from a seedpoint, a large number of pathways are propagated from the seedpoint. The direction of each next step is drawn from a distribution of possible orientations (Jones et al., 2008). Probabilistic algorithms are less dependent upon well-defined principal eigenvectors, and typically do not have an anisotropy threshold as a termination criteria, but the only stopping criterion is the angular deviation between successive steps. This facilitates the reconstruction of trajectories into and from areas of low anisotropy such as the grey matter (Behrens et al., 2003, 2007). The result of the probabilistic method is a map, which quantifies the confidence that a pathway can be found between each voxel and the seedpoint (Jones et al., 2008).

Berman et al. successfully delineated the motor and somatosensory tracts with 3D DTI fibre tracking in neonates imaged between the 28$^{th}$ and 43$^{rd}$ postmenstrual weeks. Using deterministic and probabilistic fibre tracking, all tract-specific diffusion parameters were found to be significantly correlated with age, and the motor tracts were found to have higher anisotropy and lower diffusivity than the somatosensory pathway. By segmenting the 3D fiber tracts by slice, measurements from different axial levels of the brain were found to vary with region and age (Fig. 15) (Berman et al., 2005). Using probabilistic tractography, Counsell et al. (2007) visualized and quantified connectivity distribution in a number of white matter tracts, including the corticospinal tracts, optic radiations, fibres of the genu and the splenium of the corpus callosum, superior longitudinal fasciculus, and inferior fronto-occipital fasciculus, and they mapped the distribution of fibres within the thalamus connecting to specific cortical regions. They demonstrated in 11 ex-preterm 2-year-old infants with normal development and without evidence of focal lesions on MRI that connections to and from the thalamus showed a strong correspondence with those shown in adult human brains (Behrens et al., 2003). Connections to and from the frontal/temporal cortex project to a region including the mediodorsal nucleus, connections from parietal/occipital cortex project to the pulvinar, connections from the motor area project to ventrolateral nuclei and those from the somatosensory area project to the ventral posterior nucleus. However, investigating one further child with a large right-sided porencephalic cyst secondary to previous periventricular haemorrhagic infarction showed diminished thalamo-cortical projections on the side ipsilateral to the porencephalic cyst (Fig. 16) (Counsell et al., 2007).

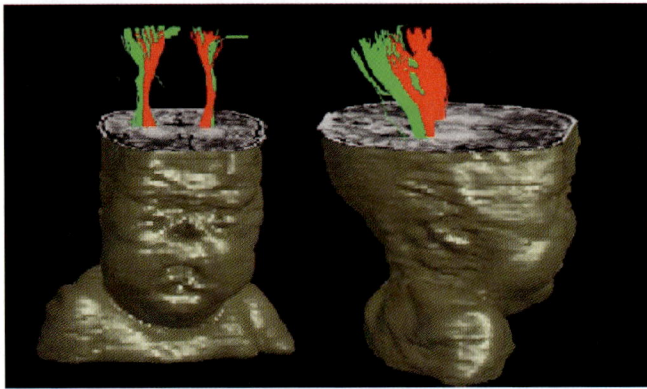

*Fig. 15. Motor and sensory tracts (Berman* et al.*, 2005).*

*Chapter 4 Diffusion MR techniques to study the neonatal brain*

Bassi *et al.* (2008) delineated the optic radiations in 37 preterm infants at term-equivalent age using probabilistic tractography. Visual function was tested using a battery assessing different aspects of visual abilities (Ricci *et al.*, 2007a, 2007b). FA values of the tracts generated from a seed mask placed in the white matter lateral to the lateral geniculate nucleus were also determined and examined using TBSS, identifying significant linear correlation between visual assessment scores and FA in the optic radiations.

## Future developments and applications

### Foetal DWI

Several studies have now used DWI to assess the brain of the preterm infant at term-equivalent age. This has highlighted differences in *ex utero* development of the immature brain. In these studies term-born infants have acted as controls. This is not ideal for following the developmental processes between 23 and 40 weeks. The ideal control would be to study the brain

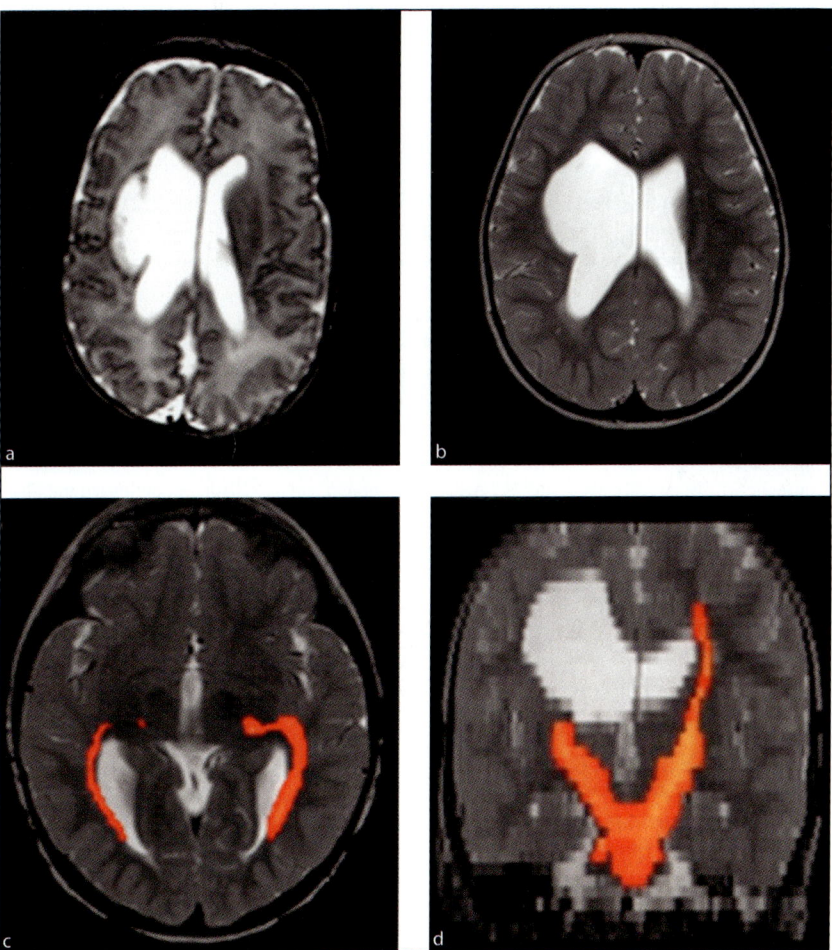

*Fig. 16. Right-sided porencephalic cyst at child at term (**a**) and at 2-year of age (**b**) on conventional MRI. Optic radiation (**c**) and corticospinal tracts (**d**) are shown (Counsell et al., 2007).*

developing *in utero* with foetal MRI. Fetal MRI is mainly used to confirm or detect abnormalities suspected on antenatal ultrasound. Early reports using DWI included study of the normal foetal brain (Baldoli *et al.*, 2002) and one of an abnormal foetus (Righini *et al.*, 2004). Foetal DWI is challenging because of the effects of foetal motion; in some centers successful DWI of the foetus is only obtained in the presence of maternal sedation. It does have promise as a tool for assessing early ischaemic change in the foetal brain either in association with a possible injury (*e.g.*, maternal trauma or in high-risk pregnancies where ischaemia may occur as a complication, as in the case of monochorionic twins) (McKinstry *et al.*, 2002). A recent approach uses dynamic acquisition to acquire DTI in 16 directions, producing high-signal-to-noise, high-resolution ADC maps and acceptable FA maps (Jiang *et al.*, 2007). A recent study has produced 18-direction DTI data for the foetus between 18–37 weeks' gestation, but no motion correction was used (Kasprian *et al.*, 2008).

## Imaging at 3T

Imaging at 3T opens up possibilities for improving signal to noise in neonatal imaging. This may be used to shorten examination times. For diffusion sequences, imaging at 3T allows sufficient signal to noise to increase b-values to more than 1,000 mm$^2$/s.

## References

Allen, M.C. (2008): Neurodevelopmental outcome of preterm infants. *Curr. Opin. Neurol.* **21**, 123–128.

Anjari, M., Srinivasan, L., Allsop, J.M., Hajnal, J.V., Rutherford, M.A., Edwards, A.D. & Counsell, S.J. (2007): Diffusion tensor imaging with tract-based spatial statistics reveals local white matter abnormalities in preterm infants. *Neuroimage* **35**, 1021–1027.

Anjari, M., Counsell, S.J., Srinivasan, L., Allsop, J.M., Hajnal, J.V., Rutherford, M.A. & Edwards, A.D. (2009): The association of lung disease with cerebral white matter abnormalities in preterm infants. *Pediatrics* **124**, 268–276.

Arzoumanian, Y., Mirmiran, M., Barnes, P.D., *et al.* (2003): Diffusion tensor brain imaging findings at term–equivalent age may predict neurologic abnormalities in low birth weight preterm infants. *AJNR Am. J. Neuroradiol.* **24**, 1646–1653.

Baldoli, C., Righini, A., Parazzini, C., Scotti, G. & Triulzi, F. (2002): Demonstration of acute ischaemic lesions in the fetal brain by diffusion magnetic resonance imaging. *Ann. Neurol.* **52**, 243–246.

Ball, G., Counsell, S.J., Anjari, M., Merchant, N., Arichi, T., Doria, V., *et al.* (2010): An optimised tract-based spatial statistics protocol for neonates: applications to prematurity and chronic lung disease. *Neuroimage* **53**, 94–102.

Barkovich, A.J. (1992): MR and CT evaluation of profound neonatal and infantile asphyxia. *Am. J. Neuroradiol.* **13**, 959–972.

Barkovich, A.J., Westmark, K.D., Bedi, H.S., Partridge, J.C., Ferriero, D.M. & Vigneron, D.B. (2001): Proton spectroscopy and diffusion imaging on the first day of life after perinatal asphyxia: preliminary report. *Am. J. Neuroradiol.* **22**, 1786–1794.

Barkovich, A.J., Miller, S.P., Bartha, A., Newton, N., Hamrick, S.E., Mukherjee, P., *et al.* (2006): MR imaging, MR spectroscopy, and diffusion tensor imaging of sequential studies in neonates with encephalopathy. *AJNR Am. J. Neuroradiol.* **27**, 533–547.

Barnerias, C., Boddaert, N., Pascale, G., Isabelle, D., Hertz Pannier, L., Dulac, O., *et al.* (2008): Unusual magnetic resonance imaging features in Menkes disease. *Brain Dev.* **30**, 489–492.

Bartha, A.I., Yap, K.R., Miller, S.P., Jeremy, R.J., Nishimoto, M., Vigneron, D.B., *et al.* (2007): The normal neonatal brain: MR imaging, diffusion tensor imaging, and 3D MR spectroscopy in healthy term neonates. *AJNR Am. J. Neuroradiol.* **28**, 1015–1021.

Bassi, L., Ricci, D., Volzone, A., Allsop, J.M., Srinivasan, L., Pai, A., *et al.* (2008): Probabilistic diffusion tractography of the optic radiations and visual function in preterm infants at term equivalent age. *Brain* **131**, 573–582.

Behrens, T.E., Johansen-Berg, H., Woolrich, M.W., Smith, S.M., Wheeler-Kingshott, C.A. & Boulby, P.A. (2003): Noninvasive mapping of connections between human thalamus and cortex using diffusion imaging. *Nat. Neurosci.* **6**, 750–757.

Behrens, T.E., Johansen-Berg, H., Jbabdi, S., Rushworth, M.F. & Woolrich, M.W. (2007): Probabilistic diffusion tractography with multiple fibre orientations: what can we gain? *Neuroimage* **34**, 144–155.

Berman, J.I., Mukherjee, P., Partridge, S.C., Miller, S.P., Ferriero, D.M., Barkovich, A.J., et al. (2005): Quantitative diffusion tensor MRI fiber tractography of sensorimotor white matter development in premature infants. *Neuroimage* **27**, 862–871.

Besser, P.J. & Pierpaoli, C. (1994): Microstructural and physiological features of tissues elucidated by quantitative diffusion-tensor MRI. *J. Magn. Reson.* **B103**, 247–254.

Boichot, C., Walker, P.M., Durand, C., Grimaldi, M., Chapuis, S., Gouyon, J.B. & Brunotte, F. (2006): Term neonate prognoses after perinatal asphyxia: contributions of MR imaging, MR spectroscopy, relaxation times, and apparent diffusion coefficients. *Radiology* **239**, 839–848.

Burdette, J.H. & Elster, A.D. (2002): Diffusion-weighted imaging of cerebral infarctions: are higher values better? *J. Comput. Assist. Tomogr.* **26**, 622–627.

Cavalleri, F., Berardi, A., Burlina, A.B., Ferrari, F. & Mavilla, L. (2002): Diffusion-weighted MRI of maple syrup urine disease encephalopathy. *Neuroradiology* **44**, 499–502.

Counsell, S.J., Allsop, J.M., Harrison, M.C., Larkma, D.J., Kennea, N.L., Kapellou, O., et al. (2003): Diffusion-weighted imaging of the brain in preterm infants with focal and diffuse white matter abnormality. *Pediatrics* **112**, 1–7.

Counsell, S.J., Shen, Y., Boardman, J.P., Larkman, D.J., Kapellou, O., Ward, P., et al. (2006): Axial and radial diffusivity in preterm infants who have diffuse white matter changes on magnetic resonance imaging at term-equivalent age. *Pediatrics* **117**, 376–386.

Counsell, S.J., Dyet, L.E., Larkman, D.J., Nunes, R.G., Boardman, J.P., Allsop, J.M., et al. (2007): Thalamo-cortical connectivity in children born preterm mapped using probabilistic magnetic resonance tractography. *Neuroimage* **34**, 896–904.

Counsell, S.J., Edwards, A.D., Chew, A.T., Anjari, M., Dyet, L.E., Srinivasan, L., et al. (2008): Specific relations between neurodevelopmental abilities and white matter microstructure in children born preterm. *Brain* **131**, 3201–3208.

Cowan, F., Dubowitz, L., Mercuri, E., Counsell, S. & Rutherford, M. (2003): White matter injury can lead to cognitive without major motor deficits in following perinatal asphyxia and early encephalopathy. *Dev. Med. Child Neurol. Suppl.* **93**, 14.

Cowan, F.M., Pennock, J.M., Hanrahan, J.D., Manji, K.P. & Edwards, A.D. (1994): Early detection of cerebral infarction and hypoxic ischaemic encephalopathy in neonates using diffusion-weighted magnetic resonance imaging. *Neuropediatrics* **25**, 172–175.

DeLano, M.C. & Cao, Y. (2002): High b-value diffusion imaging. *Neuroimag. Clin. N. Am.* **12**, 21–34.

De Vries, L.S., Groenendaal, F., van Haastert, I.C., Eken, P., Rademaker, K.J. & Meiners, L.C. (1999): Asymmetrical myelination of the posterior limb of the internal capsule in infants with periventricular haemorrhagic infarction: an early predictor of hemiplegia. *Neuropediatrics* **30**, 314–319.

De Vries, L.S., Van der Grond, J., Van Haastert, I.C. & Groenendaal, F. (2005): Prediction of outcome in new-born infants with arterial ischaemic stroke using diffusion-weighted magnetic resonance imaging. *Neuropediatrics* **36**, 12–20.

Dudink, J., Lequin, M., van Pul, C., Buijs, J., Conneman, N., van Goudoever, J. & Govaert, P. (2007): Fractional anisotropy in white matter tracts of very-low-birth-weight infants. *Pediatr. Radiol.* **37**, 1216–1223.

Dudink, J., Larkman, D.J., Kapellou, O., Boardman, J.P., Allsop, J.M., Cowan, F.M. et al. (2008): High b-value diffusion tensor imaging of the neonatal brain at 3T. *AJNR Am. J. Neuroradiol.* E-pub ahead of print Aug 7, 2008.

Fiesbach, J.B., Jansen, O., Schellinger, P.D., Heiland, S., Hacke, W. & Sartor, K. (2002): Serial analysis of the apparent diffusion coefficient time course in human stroke. *Neuroradiology* **44**, 294–298.

Forbes, K.P., Pipe, J.G. & Bird, R. (2000): Neonatal hypoxic-ischaemic encephalopathy: detection with diffusion-weighted MR imaging. *Am. J. Neuroradiol.* **21**, 1490–1496.

Forbes, K.P., Pipe, J.G. & Bird, C.R. (2002): Changes in brain water diffusion during the 1$^{st}$ year of life. *Radiology* **222**, 405–409.

Gimenez, M., Miranda, M.J., Born, A.P., Nagy, Z., Rostrup, E. & Jernigan, T.L. (2008): Accelerated white matter development in preterm infants: a voxel-base morphometry study with diffusion MR imaging. *Neur. Imag.* **41**, 728–734.

Hüppi, P.S. & Dubois, J. (2006): Diffusion tensor imaging of brain development. *Semin. Fetal Neonat. Med.* **11**, 489–497.

Hüppi, P.S., Maier, S.E. & Peled Jolesz, F.A. (1998): Microstructural development of human newborn cerebral white matter assessed in vivo by diffusion tensor magnetic resonance imaging. *Pediatr. Res.* **44**, 584–590.

Hüppi, P.S., Murphy, B., Maier, S.E., Zientara, G.P., Inder, T.E., Barnes, P.D., et al. (2001): Microstructural brain development after perinatal cerebral white matter injury assessed by diffusion tensor magnetic resonance imaging. *Pediatrics* **107**, 455–460.

Inder, T., Hüppi, P.S., Zientara, G.P., Maier, S.E., Jolesz, F.A., di Salvo, D., et al. (1999): Early detection of periventricular leukomalacia by diffusion-weighted magnetic resonance imaging techniques. *J. Pediatr.* **134**, 631–634.

Jaermann, T., Crelier, G., Pruessmann, K.P., Golay, X., Netsch, T., Van Muiswinkel, A.M., et al. (2004): SENSE-DTI at 3T. *Magn. Reson. Med.* **51**, 230–236.

Jiang, S., Xue, H., Counsell, S., Anjari, M., Allsop, J., Rutherford, M., et al. (2007): In-utero three dimension high resolution fetal brain diffusion tensor imaging. *Med. Image Comput. Comput. Assist Interv.* **10**, 18–26.

Jones, D.K. (2008): Studying connections in the living human brain with diffusion MRI. *Cortex* **44**, 936–952.

Kasprian, G., Brugger, P.C., Weber, M., Krssák, M., Krampl, E., Herold, C. & Prayer, D. (2008): *In utero* tractography of fetal white matter development. *Neuroimage* **43**, 213–224.

Khong, P.L., Lam, B.C., Chung, B.H., Wong, K.Y. & Ooi, G.C. (2003): Diffusion-weighted MR imaging in neonatal nonketotic hyperglycinemia. *Am. J. Neuroradiol.* **24**, 1181–1183.

Kirton, A., Shroff, M., Visvanathan, T. & deVeber, G. (2007): Quantified corticospinal tract diffusion restriction predicts neonatal stroke outcome. *Stroke* **38**, 974–980.

Krishnamoorthy, K.S., Soman. T.B., Takeoka, M. & Schaefer, P.W. (2000): Diffusion-weighted imaging in neonatal cerebral infarction: clinical utility and follow-up. *J. Child Neurol.* **15**, 592–602.

Krishnan, M.L., Dyet, L.E., Boardman, J.P., Kapellou, O., Allsop, J.M., Cowan, F., et al. (2007): Relationship between white matter apparent diffusion coefficients in preterm infants at term-equivalent age and developmental outcome at 2 years. *Pediatrics* **120**, e604–609.

Kuenzle, C., Baenziger, O., Martin, E., Thun-Hohenstein, L., Steinlin, M., Good, M., et al. (1994): Prognostic value of early MR imaging in term infants with severe perinatal asphyxia. *Neuropediatrics* **25**, 191–200.

Kumar, R., Macey, P.M., Woo, M.A., Alger, J.R. & Harper, R.M. (2008): Diffusion tensor imaging demonstrates brainstem and cerebellar abnormalities in congenital central hypoventilation syndrome. *Pediatr. Res.* **64**, 275–280.

Larroque, B., Ancel, P.Y. & Marret, S. (2008): Neurodevelopmental disabilities and special care of 5-year-old children born before 33 weeks gestation (the EPIPAGE study): a longitudinal cohort study. *Lancet* **371**, 813–820.

Le Bihan, D., Mangin, J.F., Poupon, C., Clark, C.A., Pappata, S. & Molko, N. (2001): Diffusion tensor imaging: concepts and applications. *J. Magn. Reson. Imag.* **13**, 534–546.

Liauw, L., van der Grond, J., van den Berg-Huysmans, A.A., Palm-Meinders, I.H., van Buchem, M.A. & van Wezel-Meijler, G. (2008): Hypoxic-ischaemic encephalopathy: diagnostic value of conventional MR imaging pulse sequences in term-born neonates. *Radiology* **247**, 204–212.

Lynch, J.K. (2009): Epidemiology and classification of perinatal stroke. *Semin. Fetal Neonatal Med.* **14**, 245–249.

Mader, I., Schoning, M., Klose, U. & Kuker, W. (2002): Neonatal cerebral infarction diagnosed by diffusion-weighted MRI: pseudonormalization occurs early. *Stroke* **33**, 1142–1145.

McKinstry, R.C., Mathur, A., Miller, J.H., Ozcan, A., Snyder, A.Z., Schefft, G.L., et al. (2002): Radial organization of developing preterm human cerebral cortex revealed by non-invasive water diffusion anisotropy MRI. *Cereb. Cortex* **12**, 1237–1243.

McKinstry, R.C., Miller, J.H., Synder, A.Z., Mathur, A., Schefft, G.I. & Almli, C.R. (2002): A prospective, longitudinal diffusion tensor imaging study of brain injury in newborns. *Neurology* **59**, 824–833.

Ment, L., Hirtz, D. & Hüppi, P. (2009): Imaging biomarkers of outcome in the developing preterm brain. *Lancet Neurol.* **8**, 1042–1045.

Mercuri, E., Rutherford, M., Cowan, F., Azzopardi, D., Bydder, G., Pennock, J., et al. (1999): Early prognostic indicators of outcome in infants with neonatal cerebral infarction: a clinical EEG and MRI study. *Paediatrics* **103**, 39–46.

Mercuri, E., Ricci, D., Cowan, F., Lessing, D., Frisone, M., Haatja, L., et al. (2000): Head growth in infants with hypoxic-ischaemic encephalopathy: correlation with neonatal magnetic resonance imaging. *Pediatrics* **106**, 235–243.

Miller, J.H., McKinstry, R.C., Philip, J.V., Mukherjee, P. & Neil, J.J. (2003): Diffusion-tensor MR imaging of normal brain maturation: a guide to structural development and myelination. *Am. J. Roentgenol.* **180**, 851–859.

Miller, S.P., Vigneron, D.B., Henry, R.G., Bohland, M.A., Ceppi-Cozzio, C., Hoffman, C., et al. (2002): Serial quantitative diffusion tensor MRI of the premature brain: development in newborns with and without injury. *J. Magn. Reson. Imaging* **16**, 621–632.

Mori, S. & Zhang, J. (2006): Principles of diffusion tensor imaging and its applications to basic neuroscience research. *Neuron.* **51**, 527–539.

Moseley, M.E., Cohen, Y., Kucharczyk, J., Mintorovitch, J., Asgari, H.S., Wendland, M.F., et al. (1990): Diffusion-weighted MR imaging of anisotropic water diffusion in cat central nervous system. *Radiology* **176**, 439–445.

Mukherjee, P., Miller, J.H., Shimony, J.S., Philip, J.V., Nehra, D., Snyder, A.Z., et al. (2002): Diffusion-tensor MR imaging of gray and white matter development during normal human brain maturation. *Am. J. Neuroradiol.* **23**, 1445–1456.

Neubauer, A.P., Voss, W. & Kattner, E. (2008): Outcome of extremely low birth weight survivors at school age: the influence of perinatal parameters on neurodevelopment. *Eur. J. Paedtr.* **167**, 87–95.

Poretti, A., Boltshauser, E., Loenneker, T., Valente, E.M., Brancati, F., Il'yasov, K. & Huisman, T.A. (2007): Diffusion tensor imaging in Joubert syndrome. *AJNR Am J. Neuroradiol.* **28**, 1929–1933.

Porter, E.J., Counsell, S.J., Edwards, A.D., Allsop, J. & Azzopardi, D. (2010): Tract-based spatial statistics of magnetic resonance images to assess disease and treatment effects in perinatal asphyxial encephalopathy. *Pediatr. Res.* **68**, 205–209.

Provenzale, J.M., Liang, L., DeLong, D. & White, L.E. (2007): Diffusion tensor imaging assessment of brain white matter maturation during the first postnatal year. *AJR Am. J. Roentgenol.* **189**, 476–486.

Ricci, D., Cesarini, L., Groppo, M., De Carli, A., Gallini, F., Serrao, F., et al. (2008): Early assessment of visual function in full term newborns. *Early Hum. Dev.* **84**, 107–113.

Ricci, D., Romeo, D.M.M., Serrao, F., Cesarini, L., Gallini, F., Cota, F., et al. (2008): Application of a neonatal assessment of visual function in a population of low risk full-term newborn. *Early Hum. Dev.* **84**, 277–280.

Righini, A., Salmona. S., Bianchini. E., Zirpoli, S., Moschetta, M., Kustermann, A., et al. (2004): Prenatal magnetic resonance imaging evaluation of ischaemic brain lesions in the survivors of monochorionic twin pregnancies: report of 3 cases. *J. Comput. Assist. Tomogr.* **28**, 87–92.

Roelants-van Rijn, A.M., Nikkels, P.G., Groenendaal, F., van Der Grond, J., Barth, P.G., Snoeck, I., et al. (2001): Neonatal diffusion-weighted MR imaging: relation with histopathology or follow-up MR examination. *Neuropediatrics* **32**, 286–294.

Rutherford, M.A. (2002): *MRI of the Neonatal Brain*. Philadelphia, PA: W.B. Saunders.

Rutherford, M.A., Pennock, J.M., Schwieso, J.E., Cowan, F.M. & Dubowitz, L.M.S. (1996): Hypoxic-ischaemic encephalopathy: early and late MRI findings and clinical outcome. *Arch. Dis. Child.* **75**, 145–151.

Rutherford, M.A., Pennock, J.M., Cowan, F.M., Dubowitz, L.M., Hajnal, J.V. & Bydder, G.M. (1997a): Does the brain regenerate after perinatal infarction? *Eur. J. Paediatr. Neurol.* **1**, 13–17.

Rutherford, M.A., Pennock, J.M., Cowan, F.M., Saeed, N., Hajnal, J.V. & Bydder, G.M. (1997b): Detection of subtle changes in the brains of infants and children via subvoxel registration and subtraction of serial MR imag's. *Am. J. Neuroradiol.* **18**, 829–835.

Rutherford, M.A., Pennock, J.M., Counsell, S.J., Mercuri, E., Cowan, F.M., Dubowitz, L.M. & Edwards, A.D. (1998): Abnormal magnetic resonance signal in the internal capsule predicts poor neurodevelopmental outcome in infants with hypoxic-ischaemic encephalopathy. *Pediatrics* **102**, 323–328.

Rutherford, M.A., Counsell, S.J., Allsop, J., Boardman, J., Kapeloou, O., Larkman, D., et al. (2004): Diffusion weighted MR imaging in perinatal brain injury: a comparison with site of lesion and time from birth. *Pediatrics* **114**, 1004–1014.

Rutherford, M.A., Ward, P., Allsop, J., Malamatentiou, C. & Counsell, S. (2005): Magnetic resonance imaging in neonatal encephalopathy. *Early Hum. Dev.* **81**, 13–25.

Saigal, S. & Doyle, L.W. (2008): An overview of mortality and sequel of preterm birth from infancy till adulthood. *Lancet* **371**, 261–269.

Shah, D.K., Tingay, D.G., Fink, A.M., Hunt, R.W. & Dargaville, P.A. (2005): Magnetic resonance imaging in neonatal nonketotic hyperglycinemia. *Pediatr. Neurol.* **33**, 50–52.

Smith, S.M., Jenkinson, M., Johansen-Berg, H., Rueckert, D., Nichols, T.E., Mackay, C.E., et al. (2006): Tract-based spatial statistics: voxelwise analysis of multi-subject diffusion data. *Neuroimage* **31**, 1487–1505.

Sreenan, C., Bhargava, R. & Robertson, C.M. (2000): Cerebral infarction in the term newborn: clinical presentation and long-term outcome. *J. Pediatr.* **137**, 351–355.

Stejskal, E.O. & Tanner, J.E. (1965): Spin diffusion measurements: spin echos in the presence of a time-dependent field gradient. *J. Chem. Phys.* **42**, 288–292.

Takeoka, M., Soman, T.B., Yoshii, A., Caviness, V.S., Jr., Gonzalez, R.G., Grant, P.E. & Krishnamoorthy, K.S. (2002): Diffusion-weighted images in neonatal cerebral hypoxic-ischaemic injury. *Pediatr. Neurol.* **26**, 274–281.

Tanner, S.F., Ramenghi, L.A., Ridgway, J.P., Berry, E., Saysell, M.A., Martine, D., et al. (2000): Quantitative comparison of intrabrain diffusion in adults and preterm and term neonates and infants. *Am. J. Roentgenol.* **174**, 1643–1649.

Vermeulen, R.J., Fetter, W.P., Hendrikx, L., Van Schie, P.E., van der Knaap, M.S. & Barkhof, F. (2003): Diffusion-weighted MRI in severe neonatal hypoxic-ischaemia: the white cerebrum. *Neuropediatrics* **34**, 72–76.

Vermeulen, R.J., van Schie, P.E., Hendrikx, L., Barkhof, F., van Weissenbruch, M., Knol, D.L. & Pouwels, P.J. (2008): Diffusion-weighted and conventional MR imaging in neonatal hypoxic ischaemia: two-year follow-up study. *Radiology* **249,** 63163–9.

Voss, W., Neubauer, A.P., Wachtendorf, M., Verhey, J.F. & Kattner, E. (2007): Neurodevelopmental outcome in extremely low birth weight infants: what is the minimum age for reliable prognosis? *Acta Pediat.* **96,** 342–147.

Ward, P., Counsell, S., Allsop, J., Cowan, F., Shen, Y., Edwards, D. & Rutherford, M. (2006): Reduced fractional anisotropy on diffusion tensor magnetic resonance imaging after hypoxic-ischaemic encephalopathy. *Pediatrics* **117,** e619–e630.

Winter, J.D., Lee, D.S., Hung, R.M., Levin, S.D., Rogers, J.M., Thompson, R.T. & Gelman, N. (2007): Apparent diffusion coefficient pseudonormalization time in neonatal hypoxic-ischaemic encephalopathy. *Pediatr. Neurol.* **37,** 255–262.

Wolf, R.L., Zimmerman, R.A., Clancy, R. & Haselgrove, J.H. (2001): Quantitative apparent diffusion coefficient measurements in term neonates for early detection of hypoxic-ischaemic brain injury: initial experience. *Radiology* **218,** 825–833.

Zarifi, M.K., Astrakas, L.G., Poussaint, T.Y., Plessis, A., Zurakowski, D. & Tzika, A.A. (2002): Prediction of adverse outcome with cerebral lactate level and apparent diffusion coefficient in infants with perinatal asphyxia. *Radiology* **225,** 859–870.

Chapter 5

# Visual development: new tools for assessment in the neonatal period

Daniela Ricci*, Domenico M. Romeo*º and Eugenio Mercuri*

*Paediatric Neurology Unit, Catholic University, Rome, Italy;
ºDivision of Child Neurology and Psychiatry, Department of Paediatrics,
University of Catania, Italy
daniricciola@libero.it

## Summary

We report the development of a simple protocol for the assessment of different aspects of visual function in the neonatal period that can easily be performed in infants at risk of developing visual and neurologic abnormalities.

The protocol includes nine items assessing a number of different aspects of visual function, ranging from ocular movements to reaction to coloured targets, and discrimination of stripes with increasing spatial frequency or attention at distance. This battery can be used even before 35 weeks' postmenstrual age (PMA), but not reliably before 31 weeks' postmenstrual age. The application of this tool to large cohorts of both term-born infants and preterm infants at 35 and 40 weeks' PMA allowed the collection of age-specific normative data that can be used as reference data.

## Introduction

In the last decades considerable advances have been made in the understanding of the development of vision in the first years of life. This has mainly been due to the increased availability of early neuroimaging and to the development of age-specific tests assessing different aspects of visual function (Atkinson *et al.*, 1979, 1993; van Hof-van Duin, 1986). The possibility of assessing different aspects of visual function including acuity, visual fields, attention at distance, and fixation shift have allowed us to establish that different aspects of visual function develop at different ages, reflecting the maturation of different cortical areas.

In contrast, the assessment of visual function in the neonatal period, although included in most neonatal neurologic assessments, has mainly been limited to the evaluation of the ability to fix and follow a specific target (Amiel-Tison & Gosselin, 2001; Dubowitz *et al.*, 1998). Since the 1980s it has been reported that fixing and tracking can be elicited as early as 30–32 weeks' gestation and that the responses become more complete as the age gets closer to term-equivalent age (Dubowitz *et al.*, 1980; Miranda, 1970; Morante *et al.*, 1982). These responses, however,

55

can be elicited even in neonates with major brain lesions, as these functions in the neonatal period are mediated by subcortical pathways (Dubowitz *et al.*, 1986). Consequently, a more comprehensive assessment is also needed, including other aspects of neonatal visual function.

In this chapter we will review our work on the neonatal assessment of visual function, including the development of a structured protocol for the assessment of different aspects of neonatal visual function and its application to term and preterm infants and to neonates with lesions.

## Early assessment of visual function in full-term newborns

In developing our examination protocol, we aimed to assess different aspects of visual function already in the first days after birth, not only in infants born at term, but also in preterm infants before term-equivalent age. We therefore aimed to develop a structured protocol that would be:

– 1. reliable;
– 2. short (not longer than 5 minutes);
– 3. easy to perform;
– 4. requiring small equipment that is easy to clean;
– 5. easy to use in difficult situations [*e.g.*, Neonatal Intensive Care Unit (NICU) incubators].

A number of items were selected, after reviewing the literature on neonatal visual abilities, on the most appropriate specific targets, and on their applicability in incubators (Amiel-Tison & Gosselin, 2001; Brazelton *et al.*, 1986; Dobson & Teller, 1978; Dobson *et al.*, 1987; Dubowitz *et al.*, 1980; Miranda, 1970; Morante *et al.*, 1982; Dubowitz *et al.*, 1998; Fantz, 1963; Sigman *et al.*, 1973).

The original *pro forma* included a variety of items ranging from assessment of ocular movement (spontaneous and with the target) and fixing and tracking with different targets, to reaction to coloured target, discrimination of stripes with increasing spatial frequency and attention at distance (Fig. 1).

This *pro forma* was pilot-tested in a cohort of 90 full-term infants assessed at 48 hours from birth, and a final selection was made according to the feasibility of the various items, excluding those that were difficult to perform, time-consuming, or found not to be very discriminating (Ricci *et al.*, 2008a).

The remaining nine items proved to be feasible in newborns as young as 48 hours from birth, easy and short to perform in a neonatal unit or even in a neonatal intensive care unit, and having a good inter-observer reliability. The nine items explore various aspects of visual function such as the ability to fix and follow a target, and the more complex aspects of visual abilities, such as reaction to a colour target, and discrimination of black and white stripes with increasing spatial frequency and attention at distance (Fig. 2).

## Application of the neonatal assessment of visual function in a population of low-risk full-term newborn infants

This final version was validated in a cohort of 124 low-risk term-born neonates assessed at 48 hours from birth in order to provide normative data and frequency distribution for each item. The inter-observer agreement was 97 per cent (Ricci *et al.*, 2008b).

Chapter 5  New tools for assessment of visual development in the neonatal period

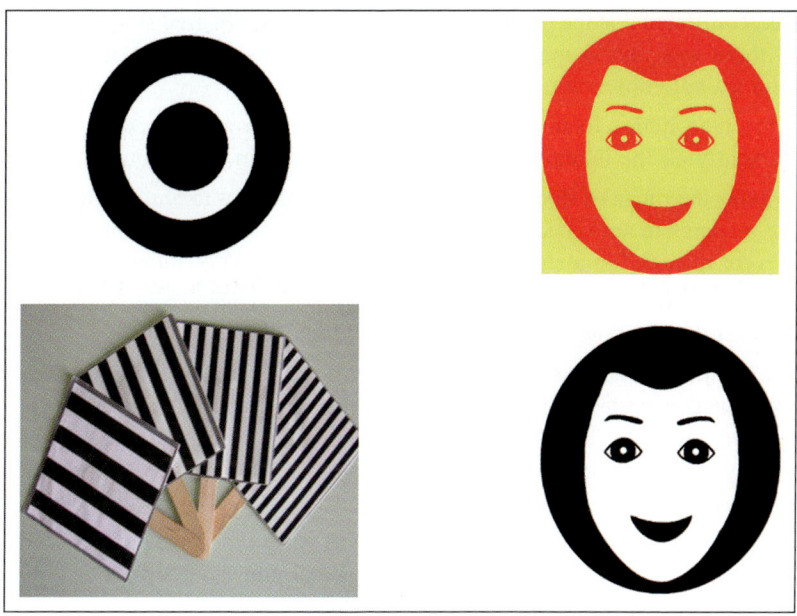

Fig. 1. Targets used for the neonatal assessment.

| # | Item | Target | | | | |
|---|------|--------|---|---|---|---|
| 1 | *Spontaneous ocular mobility:* note spontaneous ocular movements before presenting a target | | Mainly conjugated | Occasional strabismus  R  L | Occasional lateral nystagmus  R  L | Intermittent strabismus  nystagmus  R  L    R  L | Continuous strabismus  nystagmus  R  L    R  L |
| 2 | *Ocular movements with a target:* note ocular movements while presenting the target | ◎ | Mainly conjugated | Occasional strabismus  R  L | Occasional lateral nystagmus  R  L | Intermittent strabismus  nystagmus  R  L    R  L | Continuous strabismus  nystagmus  R  L    R  L |
| 3 | *Fixation:* with the target in front of the infant at 25 cm, note the ability of the infant to fix on the target | ◎ | Stable (> 3 sec) | Unstable (< 3 sec) | Absent | | |
| | **Tracking – black/white target** | | | | | | |
| | *Tracking:* note the infant's eye movement in response to the target movements | ◎ | | | | | |
| 4 | *Horizontal:* with the target at 25 cm, and starting in the midline move it slowly to both left and right | ◇ | Complete  R  L | Incomplete  R  L | Brief  R  L | Absent | |
| 5 | *Vertical:* with the target at 25 cm, and starting in the midline move it slowly upwards and downwards | ◆ | Complete  U  D | Incomplete  U  D | Brief  U  D | Absent | |
| 6 | *Arc:* with the target at 25 cm, move it slowly tracing an arc | ⬭ | Complete  R  L | Incomplete  R  L | Brief  R  L | Absent | |
| | **Colour/discrimination/attention** | | | | | | |
| 7 | *Tracking coloured stimulus* Note the infant's eye movement in response to the target movements, starting from the midline towards lateral | 🙂 | Present | Absent | | | |
| 8 | *Stripes discrimination* Note the infant's ability to fixate on a series of targets of decreasing stripe widths held at a distance of 38 cm starting with the widest stripe; note the narrowest stripe width on which the infant fixates | ▦ | Last card identified ......... | | | | |
| 9 | *Attention at distance* After eliciting central fixation move the target slowly away and a few cms laterally from the infant and note the maximal distance at which focusing is maintained | 🙂 | 0m.......... | | | | |

Fig. 2. Final pro forma *with instruction.*

The results demonstrated that the battery can be easily and reliably used at 48 hours in term-born infants, and there was only a minimal percentage of infants who did not complete the full assessment on a single observation.

In three of the nine items, fixation on a black/white and on a coloured target and tracking horizontally, nearly all the infants showed consistent results in one column.

In the other items the range of findings was wider: 73 per cent of the infants were able to track the target for a complete arc vertically and 41 per cent in a circle. Occasional abnormal ocular movements were recorded in a significant number (32 per cent) of infants.

All but one infant were able to fix on at least the first four striped cards, and all were able to keep attention on the black/white face target for at least 30 cm.

Fifty of the 124 infants have also been assessed at 72 hours from birth. In five of the nine items similar results were recorded at both 48 and 72 hours, whereas in the remaining four items (vertical and circle tracking, stripe discrimination, and attention at distance) at 72 hours there was significantly more mature response. The difference was found to be statistically significant for these four items.

These data confirm that it is possible to obtain a very early crude measure of acuity that can be easily used even in infants in incubators in a neonatal unit environment.

These results also provide information on visual abilities in a low-risk population of term-born infants and the distribution of frequency of their visual responses to our battery of visual tests. When our visual test battery is used in both clinical and research settings, these findings may be used as reference data.

## Visual function at 35 and 40 weeks' postmenstrual age in low-risk preterm infants

The same examination was used in a cohort of 109 low-risk preterm newborns (25.0 to 30.9 weeks' gestational age) assessed at 35 and 40 weeks' (term-equivalent) postmenstrual age to address the possible role of extrauterine life on the early development of visual function. Each infant was assessed twice, at 35 and at 40 weeks' postmenstrual age. The findings reported suggested that the battery for the visual function assessment was suitable for use even with preterm infants and can be easily and reliably used not only at term-equivalent age but also at 35 weeks' postmenstrual age. Preterm infants at 35 and 40 weeks were able to fix and follow in a circle, to react to a target with colour contrast, to follow a target at a distance, and to discriminate stripes of decreasing width. The findings were not related to gestational age at birth or to the presence of stage 1 or 2 ROP (retinopathy of prematurity) (Ricci *et al.*, 2008c).

Preterm infants assessed at 35 weeks' postmenstrual age were generally less mature in their visual responses than at term-equivalent age, but the differences were significant for only three items (tracking on a coloured target, attention at distance, and stripe discrimination). The comparison between the results in preterm infants and those reported in term-born infants at 48 hours from birth showed that ocular movements (spontaneous or following a target) and tracking on a black/white target vertically and in an arc were more mature in preterm infants at both 35 and 40 weeks; the abilities to fix centrally and track horizontally were not different among the three groups. These results demonstrated that early aspects of visual function may be mediated by subcortical rather than by cortical systems. The maturation of these 'subcortical' aspects of visual function could be accelerated by preterm extrauterine exposure and early extra-visual and visuomotor experiences.

Other responses (responses to colour contrast, attention at distance, and discrimination of stripes), in contrast, were less mature in preterm infants at 35 weeks compared with both preterm infants at term-equivalent age and term-born infants; these are all aspects of visual function that are likely to require some cortical input and more mature subcortical/cortical connectivity. These more cortically mediated aspects of early visual development are likely to be more dependent on postmenstrual age than on the length of extrauterine life.

## Probabilistic diffusion tractography of optic radiations and visual function in preterm infants at term-equivalent age

A subsequent study demonstrated that our neonatal visual assessment was related to an objective evaluation of the maturation of the anatomic visual pathway. We used diffusion tensor imaging (DTI) with probabilistic diffusion tractography to delineate optic radiations at term-equivalent age and compared the fractional anisotropy (FA) to a contemporaneous evaluation of visual function (Bassi *et al.*, 2008). Thirty-seven preterm infants born between 24 to 32 weeks' gestational age were examined at term-equivalent age.

Ten infants had evidence of cerebral lesions on conventional MRI.

Multiple regression analysis demonstrated that the visual findings were independently correlated with FA values, but not with gestational age at birth, postmenstrual age at scan, or the presence of lesions on conventional MRI. Visual findings appeared to be related specifically to the development of optic radiations rather than to the overall maturation of the brain, as a secondary analysis using tract-based spatial statistics to determine global brain white matter development found that only FA in the optic radiations was correlated with the results of the visual assessment.

## Early assessment of visual function in preterm infants: how early is early?

As the ability to fix and follow a target was the only visual finding reported in preterm infants as young as by 30–32 weeks' post menstrual age (PMA), we also used the neonatal battery in a cohort of low-risk infants of gestational age (GA) 25–32 weeks in order to assess the onset of other aspects of visual function (Ricci *et al.*, 2010).

If patients were reported to be clinically stable, but were not in the right behavioural state at the time of the assessment, the examiners tried to assess them later on the same day or within the same week.

Our findings suggested that a structured assessment of visual function can be reliably used only from 31 weeks onwards as only 30 per cent of infants could be assessed before 31 weeks PMA. At 31 weeks and after, surprisingly these infants were able to respond not only to the more 'basic' items such as fixation and horizontal tracking, but also to items with more structured stimuli, irrespective of the gestational age at birth.

Comparing the findings with those obtained in infants assessed at older PMA, some items (spontaneous ocular motility, fixation, tracking horizontally, and response to a coloured stimulus) were similar at 32 and 33 weeks compared to 35 weeks PMA; in the remaining items, the responses recorded at 32–33 weeks were less mature compared to those at 35 weeks, showing a progressive maturation of acuity and tracking with increasing PMA.

## Early visual assessment in preterm infants with and without brain lesions: correlation with visual and neurodevelopmental outcome at 12 months

The assessment of visual function was finally done in a cohort of infants with brain lesions affecting anatomic structures in the visual pathway as evidenced from brain imaging (Ricci *et al.*, 2011).

No systematic analysis has established the prognostic value of early visual examination in both low-risk infants and in those with brain lesions followed longitudinally from the neonatal period and at 3 and 12 months.

Using the neonatal battery in a cohort longitudinally followed and assessed with age-specific tests at the age of 1 year, we also investigated the prognostic value of the early neonatal visual assessment in preterm infants with and without brain lesions. A normal early visual assessment was a reliable indicator of normal visual function and neurodevelopment at 1 year, with fewer than 10 per cent of the infants having false-negative results and with a good sensitivity and specificity.

On the other hand, abnormal visual results at term age were less reliable indicators of visual function and neurodevelopment at 1 year. The false-positives were mainly found in infants with normal ultrasound or only minor abnormalities, and in all these, the visual assessment had normalized by 3 months; these data suggest a delayed visual maturation limited to the first 3 months.

## Conclusions

The neonatal visual assessment permits assessment of different aspects of visual function very early in life. It can be easily and reliably used in term-born and preterm infants. We suggest that this tool could be used routinely in neonatal units as part of a larger examination, including neurologic assessment, in order to collect more and specific information on the neurodevelopment of the infant. This battery can be easily performed by personnel not used to performing such visual assessment tests.

The possibility of identifying early visual deficits allows early referral of these babies to rehabilitation services where both they and their parents can get appropriate support.

**Acknowledgments:** The findings reported in this chapter are the result of a multicentre effort including our Unit and the Neonatal Unit, Catholic University, Rome; the Division of Child Neurology and Psychiatry, Department of Paediatrics, University of Catania; the Neonatal Intensive Care Unit, Department of Paediatrics, University of Catania; the Neonatal Unit, Ospedale Maggiore Policlinico, Mangiagalli, Fondazione IRCCS, Milan; the Department of Developmental Neuroscience, Stella Maris Scientific Institute, Pisa; and the Department of Paediatrics and Imaging Sciences, Hammersmith Hospital, Imperial College, London, United Kingdom. We are grateful for the support of the Mariani Foundation, Milan.

## References

Amiel-Tison, C. & Gosselin, J. (2001): *Neurological Development from Birth to Six Years: User Manual and Examination Chart*. Baltimore, Maryland: John Hopkins University Press.

Atkinson, J. & van Hof-van Duin, J. (1993): Visual assessment during the first years of life. 1993. In: *The Management of Visual Impairment in Childhood*. Publication No. 128. London: Mac Keith Press.

Atkinson, J., Braddick, O. & French, J. (1979): Contrast sensitivity of the human neonate measured by the visual evoked potential. *Invest. Ophthalmol. Vis. Sci.* **18**, 210–213.

Bassi, L., Ricci, D., Volzone, A., Allsop, J.M., Srinivasan, L., Pai, A., et al. (2008): Probabilistic diffusion tractography of the optic radiations and visual function in preterm infants at term equivalent age. *Brain* **131,** 573–582.

Brazelton, T.B., Scholl, M.L. & Robey, J.S. (1966): Visual responses in the newborn. *Pediatrics* **37,** 284–290.

Dobson, V. & Teller, D.Y. (1978): Visual acuity in human infants: a review and comparison of behavioral and electrophysiological studies. *Vision Res.* **18,** 1469–1483.

Dobson, V., Schwartz, T.L., Sandstrom, D.J. & Michel, L. (1987): Binocular visual acuity of neonates: the acuity card procedure. *Dev. Med. Child Neurol.* **29,** 199–206.

Dubowitz, L.M.S., Dubowitz. V. & Morante, A. (1980): Visual function in the newborn: a study of preterm and full-term infants. *Brain Dev.* **2,** 15–29.

Dubowitz, L.M.S., Dubowitz, V., Morante, A. & Verghote, M. (1980): Visual function in the preterm and fullterm newborn infant. *Dev. Med. Child Neurol.* **22,** 465–475.

Dubowitz, L.M., Mushin, J., de Vries, L. & Arden, G.B. (1986): Visual function in the newborn infant: is it cortically mediated? *Lancet* **1,** 1139–1141.

Dubowitz, L.M.S., Dubowitz, V. & Mercuri, E. (1998): The neurological assessment of the preterm and full-term newborn infant. In: *Textbook of Clinics in Developmental Medicine*, 2$^{nd}$ ed. Publication No. 148. London: Mac Keith Press.

Fantz, R.L. (1963): Pattern vision in newborn infant. *Science* **140,** 296–297.

Miranda, S.B. (1970): Visual abilities and pattern preferences of premature infants and full-term neonates. *J. Exp. Child Psychol.* **10,** 189–205.

Morante, A., Dubowitz, L.M.S., Levene, M. & Dubowitz, V. (1982): The development of visual function in normal and neurologically abnormal preterm and fullterm infants. *Dev. Med. Child Neurol.* **24,** 771–784.

Ricci, D., Cesarini, L., Groppo, M., De Carli, A., Gallini, F., Serrao, F., Fumagalli, M., et al. (2008a): Early assessment of visual function in full term newborns. *Early Hum. Dev.* **84,** 107–113.

Ricci, D., Romeo, D.M.M., Serrao, F., Cesarini, L., Gallini, F., Cota, F., et al. (2008b): Application of a neonatal assessment of visual function in a population of low risk full-term newborn. *Early Hum. Dev.* **84,** 277–280.

Ricci, D., Cesarini, L., Romeo, D.M., Gallini, F., Serrao, F., Groppo, M., et al. (2008c): Visual function at 35 and 40 weeks' postmenstrual age in low-risk preterm infants. *Pediatrics* **122: e,** 1193–1198.

Ricci, D., Romeo, D.M.M., Serrao, F., Gallini, F., Leone, D., Longo, M., et al. (2010): Early assessment of visual function in preterm infants: how early is early? *Early Hum. Dev.* **86,** 29–33.

Ricci, D., Romeo, D.M., Gallini, F., Groppo, M., Cesarini, L., Pisoni, S., et al. (2011): Early visual assessment in preterm infants with and without brain lesions: correlation with visual and neurodevelopmental outcome at 12 months. *Early Hum. Dev.* **87,** 177–182.

Sigman, M., Kopp, C.B., Parmelee, A.H. & Jeffrey, W.E. (1973): Visual attention and neurologic organization in neonates. *Child Dev.* **44,** 461–466.

van Hof-van Duin, J. & Mohn, G. (1986): The development of visual acuity in normal fullterm and preterm infants. *Vision Res.* **26,** 909–916.

Chapter 6

# Brain transcranial stimulation: diagnostic and therapeutic applications

Federico Ranieri, Paolo Profice, Fabio Pilato, Fioravante Capone, Lucia Florio, Michele Dileone and Vincenzo Di Lazzaro

*Institute of Neurology, Università Cattolica del Sacro Cuore, largo Francesco Vito 1, 00168 Roma, Italy*
vdilazzaro@rm.unicatt.it

## Summary

Transcranial stimulation techniques can provide relevant diagnostic information on the integrity of central motor pathways as well as important clues in the understanding of the physiology of motor systems.
Transcranial magnetic stimulation (TMS) is the most widely used technique of noninvasive brain stimulation: it activates the corticospinal tract neurons and generates motor evoked potentials (MEPs) in the muscle. MEP study allows the measurement of central motor conduction time, which can be pathologically increased in pyramidal tract lesions. However, specific considerations concern the diagnostic application of MEP study in children, especially in those under 10 years of age, because of the incomplete maturation of central motor pathways during the early stages of development.
More complex TMS protocols, based on paired-pulse stimulation, allow us to go beyond the study of the pyramidal system and can be used to evaluate the function of specific excitatory or inhibitory intracortical circuits in physiologic and pathologic conditions.
During the last several years, repetitive TMS (rTMS) and transcranial direct current stimulation (tDCS) protocols have become available that are able to induce plastic changes in the brain and to modulate the excitability of specific cortical areas for a prolonged period of time. This opens the way to the possible therapeutic application of transcranial stimulation in several neurologic or psychiatric disorders associated with abnormal excitability of specific regions of the brain or to promote recovery after brain damage.

## Overview of techniques of noninvasive brain stimulation

The introduction of new techniques for noninvasively stimulating the intact human brain has paved the way for new possibilities to study the brain function in physiologic and pathologic conditions and to diagnose and possibly treat neurologic diseases.

The first approach to the noninvasive stimulation of the brain was made by Merton and Morton (1980), who first succeeded in activating the primary motor cortex by applying transient currents to the scalp with surface electrodes. *Transcranial electrical stimulation* (TES) leads to depolarization of cortical pyramidal cells and, in turn, to activation of spinal motoneurones and muscle contraction. The overall muscle fiber depolarization can be recorded as a motor evoked potential (MEP) through surface electrodes.

In 1985, Barker and colleagues introduced a new way to stimulate the brain based on the mutual induction of electric and magnetic fields. In this technique of *transcranial magnetic stimulation* (TMS), the current flowing through a coil, positioned over the scalp surface, generates a magnetic field that in turn induces an electric field in the brain and a consequent neuronal depolarization. This prevents the painful sensation of the electric shock of TES related to the high impedance of skull and scalp tissues (Barker *et al.*, 1985).

Soon after the introduction of TMS, transcranial stimulation became an important diagnostic tool in the pathology of the pyramidal system: in the same way that motor neurography is used to study nerve conduction, the amplitude and latency of MEPs after TES or TMS can be measured to provide relevant information on the integrity of corticospinal connections (see below).

TES and TMS differ in the way they activate corticospinal cells. The data from animal experiments (Amassian *et al.*, 1987), those from single motor unit recordings (Day *et al.*, 1989), and the rare opportunity of directly recording the cortical output in humans from a spinal epidural electrode (Di Lazzaro *et al.*, 1998a) all help to shed light on the physiologic basis of the effects of transcranial stimulation. A large amount of evidence supports the view that TES activates the axons of pyramidal cells in the white matter of the brain, whereas TMS predominantly stimulates their excitatory synaptic inputs (Di Lazzaro *et al.*, 2004a). This is particularly true when the magnetic stimulus is delivered at low intensities and with a focal, figure-of-eight-shaped coil; increasing the stimulus intensity determines the direct activation of corticospinal cells (Di Lazzaro *et al.*, 1998a). The capability of TMS to activate intracortical connections led to the introduction of paired-pulse stimulation protocols, which enabled the function of specific intracortical circuits to be evaluated in physiologic (Di Lazzaro *et al.*, 1998b, 1999a; Kujirai *et al.*, 1993; Tokimura *et al.*, 1996, 2000) and pathologic conditions (Beck *et al.*, 2008; Cantello *et al.*, 2002; Di Lazzaro *et al.*, 2002a, 2006, 2007, 2008; Mhalla *et al.*, 2010; Vucic *et al.*, 2008).

More recently, technical advances made it possible to deliver trains of magnetic stimuli, with a frequency of up to 100 Hz. This kind of stimulation is referred to as *repetitive TMS* (rTMS). Repeated activation of cortical synapses, even with a stimulation intensity below the threshold for evoking motor responses, can produce a long-lasting modulation of cortical excitability of up to one hour: this effect has been related to the phenomenon of long-term potentiation/depression (LTP/LTD) of synaptic activity, and its direction and duration critically depend on rTMS frequency and intensity (see Fitzgerald *et al.*, 2006 and Hoogendam *et al.*, 2010 for a review). Another means of noninvasive modulation of brain plasticity is *transcranial direct current stimulation* (tDCS). After the capability of DCS to modulate spontaneous and evoked neuronal activity was first shown in animal preparations (Bindman *et al.*, 1962; Creutzfeld *et al.*, 1962; Purpura & McMurtry, 1965; Terzuolo & Bullock, 1956), this technique has recently been introduced as a tool to stimulate noninvasively the intact human brain (Nitsche & Paulus, 2000; Priori *et al.*, 1998; see Nitsche *et al.*, 2008 for a review). The relatively long-lasting duration of the after-effects of both rTMS and tDCS protocols opens the door to possible therapeutic application of these techniques to counteract the imbalance of excitatory and inhibitory phenomena in the brain that accompany many neurologic and psychiatric disorders.

## Diagnostic applications

The main diagnostic application of TMS is the study of *motor evoked potentials* (MEPs). These are usually recorded from upper and lower limb muscles after a cortical magnetic stimulus delivered through a circular nonfocal coil, activating the fast-conducting corticospinal projections. The difference between the latency of this response and that of the response evoked by paravertebral magnetic stimulation of the brachial or lumbosacral plexus provides information on central motor conduction time (CMCT) (Fig. 1).

Potentially any disease affecting motor cortical projections in the white matter of the brain, brainstem, or spinal cord can determine a pathologic increase of CMCT. In fact, pathologic disorders directly involving the motor pathways or lesions at brainstem or spinal cord level more likely affect CMCT. Indeed, a MEP study has a different sensitivity and specificity in different neurologic disorders (Di Lazzaro et al., 1999b). On the basis of our data from a prospective study of 1,023 patients, the higher sensitivity values of MEPs were demonstrated in spinal cord disorders (85 per cent), hereditary spastic paraplegia (80 per cent), and motor neuron diseases (74 per cent) (Fig. 2). The higher percentages of subclinical abnormalities were found in motor neuron disorders (26 per cent), muscular diseases (24 per cent), multiple sclerosis (13.5 per cent), and spinal cord diseases (12.5 per cent). The higher false-negative rates were found in sylvian stroke (36 per cent) and hereditary spastic paraplegia (16 per cent).

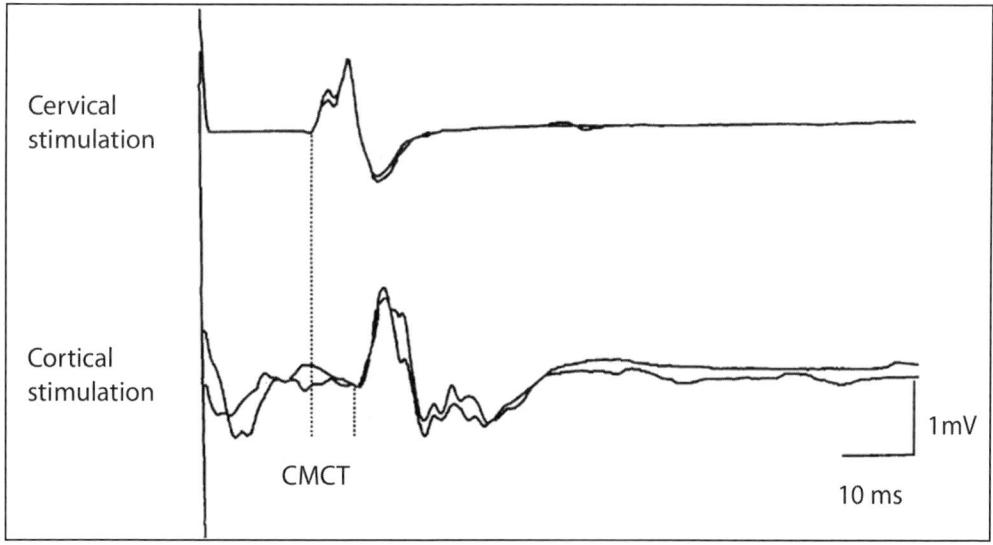

Fig. 1. Motor evoked potentials (MEPs) obtained after cortical and cervical paravertebral stimulation in the abductor digiti minimi muscle. Central motor conduction time (CMCT) is calculated as the difference between the latency of the cortical and paravertebral stimulation responses. (Modified from Di Lazzaro et al., 1999b).

A more accurate calculation of CMCT, excluding from it the radicular conduction time, is performed by subtracting the peripheral conduction time estimated from F-wave recording from the latency of cortical MEP: this allows precise determination of corticospinal conduction time. In fact, central conduction study using magnetic paravertebral stimulation, but not using the F-wave method, resulted in 12 per cent and 10 per cent of false-positive values in lower limb multiradiculopathies and in neuropathies, respectively, indicating that the F-wave method should be considered as the gold standard for central conduction determination in patients with lower motor neurone involvement (Di Lazzaro et al., 1999b, 2004b).

Specific considerations must be kept in mind when using MEP studies in paediatric age patients. As reviewed by Garvey and Mall (2008), children under 10 years of age have higher MEP thresholds, and it may even be impossible to elicit responses with the muscle at rest in children

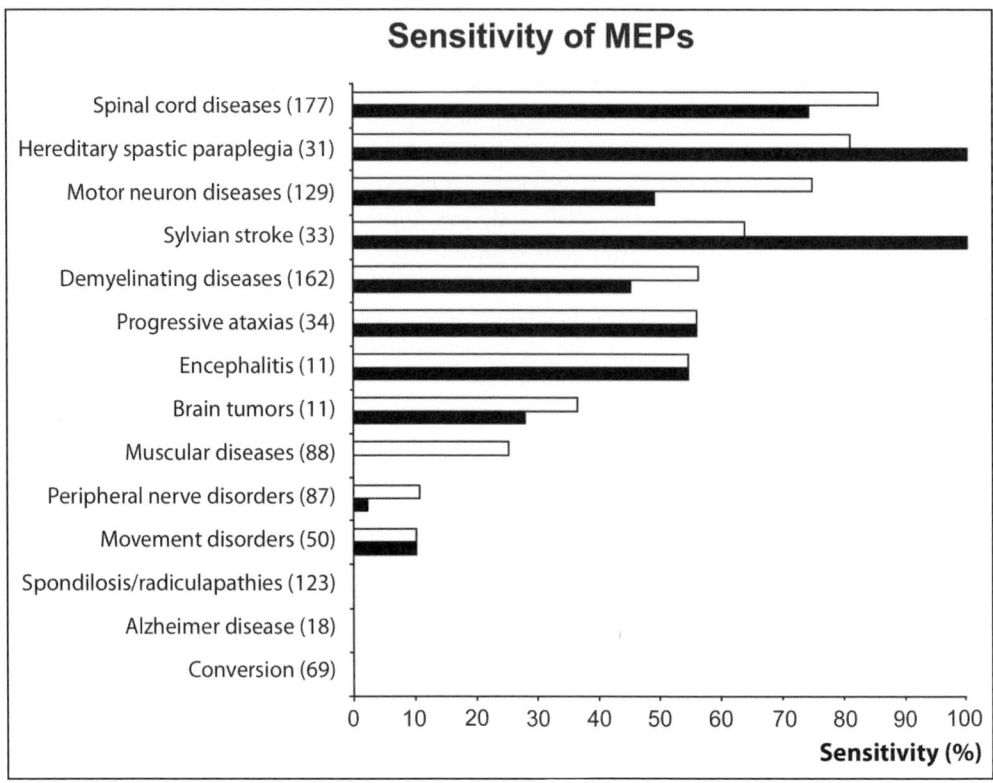

Fig. 2. Sensitivity of motor evoked potentials (MEPs, open bars) and of clinical examination (filled bars) in demonstrating corticospinal tract abnormalities in different neurologic disorders. The number of examined patients for each disorder is reported in parentheses. (Modified from Di Lazzaro et al., 1999b).

under 6 years of age. As far as MEP latency is concerned, CMCT measured during muscle contraction (active CMCT) is usually shorter than CMCT measured with the muscle at rest (resting CMCT), presumably because of recruitment of faster pyramidal tract neurons. Since active CMCT reaches maturity within the first 3–5 years of postnatal life, whereas resting CMCT does not reach maturity until early adolescence, the 'latency jump', that is, the difference between the latency of active and resting MEP, is much greater in children than in adults. Synaptic maturation within the motor cortex and central myelination have been proposed as possible mechanisms for the gradual decrease of MEP latency in developing children (Caramia et al., 1993). These considerations must be taken into account when using MEP study as a diagnostic tool in children, and appropriate normative data are necessary.

Focal TMS can be used to map the cortical representation of specific muscles. *Cortical representation maps* are obtained by measuring MEP amplitude after stimulation at a number of different scalp sites. One study examined cortical maps for several upper and lower limb muscles in typically developing children, between 6 and 14 years of age and in patients with cerebral palsy (Maegaki et al., 1999). The authors found that, in normal subjects, cortical representation of muscles respected the organization of primary motor cortex in adults (lower limb muscles more medial and upper limb muscles more lateral), indicating that the mature motor homunculus is established early in life. They also observed that ipsilateral responses were more common among cerebral palsy patients than in controls, especially when TMS was delivered to the less-damaged hemisphere of patients with marked asymmetries in brain damage, suggesting that ipsilateral motor pathways are reinforced in cerebral palsy (Maegaki et al., 1999). We recently described the case of a 14 year-old epileptic patient with hemiplegic cerebral palsy (Pilato et al., 2009) in which TMS revealed the presence of consistent ipsilateral projections from the unaffected hemisphere; this information was very useful in guiding the decision to perform hemispherectomy to treat the patient's drug-resistant epilepsy and it was predictive of good clinical outcome. In similar cases we suggest that TMS may represent a strong support to fMRI data to confirm the participation of the unaffected hemisphere in ipsilateral motor control.

The above data also suggest that cortical function is more easily reshaped during development than in adulthood, possibly because of reduced inhibitory processes. Two TMS paradigms have been used in children to assess cortical inhibitory activity: the *short-latency intracortical inhibition* (SICI) and the *ipsilateral silent period* (iSP).

SICI is a paired-pulse TMS paradigm, consisting of a subthreshold conditioning stimulus preceding by 2–3 ms the test stimulus over the primary motor cortex (Kujirai et al., 1993): the conditioning stimulus inhibits the response to the test stimulus by acting on intracortical circuits mainly through GABA-A receptors (Di Lazzaro et al., 2000). Studies comparing SICI in subjects of different ages (Mall et al., 2004; Walther et al., 2009) revealed that it is much more pronounced in adults than in children: reduced levels of SICI might reflect reduced cortical inhibition and can be associated with increased practice-dependent plasticity (Ziemann et al., 2001).

SP is a period of reduced EMG activity during sustained voluntary contraction following a suprathreshold cortical stimulus, occurring in muscles both ipsilateral and contralateral to the side of stimulation. The origin of iSP is not completely defined, but it is thought to result from the inhibitory activity of transcallosal projections on the contralateral motor cortex (Trompetto et al., 2004). ISP is absent in children under 6 years of age (Heinen et al., 1998) and progressively reduces in latency and increases in duration until about 20 years (Garvey et al., 2003).

Reduced cortical inhibitory processes might be a correlate of increased neuronal plasticity during development. However, the appropriate regulation of synapse formation and activity is crucial for normal maturation and functioning of the central nervous system and an altered homeostatic control of these processes can turn into pathology. Dystonic syndromes are one of the most studied conditions of abnormal plasticity (Quartarone et al., 2003, 2006). The plastic properties of the brain can be investigated using prolonged stimulation protocols (rTMS, tDCS) that are known to determine long-lasting effects on cortical excitability in normal subjects. In a recent study, Dileone et al. (2010) investigated the effect of a conditioning paired associative stimulation (PAS) protocol, in which ulnar nerve stimuli are followed by TMS pulses to the contralateral cortical hand area, on cortical excitability to single pulse TMS in five patients with the Costello syndrome. The Costello syndrome is a rare disorder caused by germline mutations in the *HRAS* gene, which is involved in the protein synthesis–dependent mechanisms of maintenance of LTP of synaptic activity. The specific TMS protocol used to induce cortical plasticity, combined with the recording of MEPs to single-pulse TMS, was very useful in confirming the supposed enhanced activity-dependent facilitation of cortical excitability in Costello patients (about four times greater than in controls), suggesting an increased susceptibility of synapses to undergo LTP in this pathologic condition.

## Prospective therapeutic applications

Specific protocols of transcranial stimulation can be used to modulate synaptic function through repeated activation, as in the case of repetitive TMS (rTMS), or primarily affecting the neurone resting membrane potential, as in the case of transcranial direct current stimulation (tDCS).

RTMS and tDCS protocols usually have a duration of between less than 1 and 30 minutes and can produce after-effects lasting in most cases from a few minutes to up to one hour (Hoogendam et al., 2010; Zaghi et al., 2010).

Overall, experimental data suggest that low-frequency rTMS (i.e., 1 Hz or less) produces an LTD-like effect reducing motor cortical excitability to single-pulse TMS, while high-frequency rTMS (5 Hz or more) has an LTP-like effect increasing cortical excitability (see Fitzgerald et al., 2006, for a review). More complex patterns of rTMS, such as the theta burst stimulation paradigm (Huang et al., 2005) or the paired associative stimulation (Stefan et al., 2000), produce specific effects on cortical excitability, which can be enhanced or reduced, depending on the temporal pattern of stimulation. Also, tDCS can determine a bidirectional modulation of cortical excitability that is facilitated by anodal and reduced by cathodal stimulation (Nitsche & Paulus, 2000).

The above techniques of stimulation have a potential therapeutic role in diseases of the central nervous system associated with abnormal brain excitability. In fact, in the last 15 years they have been tested in several neurologic and psychiatric disorders such as stroke, epilepsy, movement disorders, chronic pain, depression, and schizophrenia, with some encouraging results (reviewed in Fregni & Pascual-Leone, 2007). The common rationale for the application of transcranial stimulation in all these disorders is always to obtain, as a final effect, an increase in brain excitability where it is reduced or a decrease in specific areas of the brain where it is pathologically enhanced. However, it must be kept in mind that the impaired brain functions accompanied by altered excitability usually depend on a complex circuitry across more than one brain structure, and it would be optimistic to hope to restore function by simply counteracting the abnormally increased or decreased excitability of a single cortical area. Nonetheless rTMS has been shown to affect intracortical GABAergic circuit activity (Di Lazzaro et al., 2002): the amount of change is comparable to that obtained after GABAergic drug administration, even if in the opposite direction (Di Lazzaro et al., 2000), suggesting that some transcranial stimulation protocols might have a functional effect on specific intracortical systems comparable to that of commonly used drugs.

Moreover the potential therapeutic application of rTMS/tDCS protocols does not simply aim at counteracting altered excitability, but, more importantly, at reestablishing the imbalanced activity of different regions of the brain. An imbalance of the two hemispheres is exactly what occurs after stroke, where the reduced excitability of the affected hemisphere is accompanied by an increased excitability of the contralateral hemisphere, probably because of an impairment of the mechanisms of transcallosal inhibition: a maladaptive change that can oppose recovery. On this basis some therapeutic trials in stroke applied either a facilitatory stimulation protocol to the affected motor cortex or an inhibitory protocol to the contralateral one (reviewed in Hummel & Cohen, 2006).

This is also the case of an electrophysiologic study in paediatric stroke (Kirton et al., 2008), where the authors applied inhibitory rTMS to the affected motor cortex and obtained an increased MEP amplitude and interhemispheric inhibition from the affected side.

Another potential therapeutic implication of transcranial stimulation is that it may not only induce plastic changes when delivered alone, but also have a metaplastic effect by potentiating the response to a subsequent intervention based on neural plasticity, such as physiotherapy in stroke or other neurologic disorders (Baker *et al.*, 2010; Chang *et al.*, 2010; Emara *et al.*, 2010; Khedr *et al.*, 2005). In particular, given the physiologic basis of the effects of tDCS, which mainly act by modulating membrane polarization without generating action potentials, the metaplastic effect could be the main mechanism for the possible therapeutic application of this technique of stimulation.

In dystonic syndromes, which are frequent in the paediatric age group, abnormal plasticity may occur (Edwards *et al.*, 2006; Gilio *et al.*, 2007; Quartarone *et al.*, 2006), and some therapeutic attempts have been focused on restoring intracortical inhibition in the primary motor cortex (Siebner *et al.*, 1999) or inhibition from premotor areas to primary motor cortex (Huang *et al.*, 2010; Mylius *et al.*, 2009).

## References

Amassian, V.E., Stewart, M., Quirk, G.J. & Rosenthal, J.L. (1987): Physiological basis of motor effects of a transient stimulus to cerebral cortex. *Neurosurgery* **20**, 74–93.

Baker, J.M., Rorden, C. & Fridriksson, J. (2010): Using transcranial direct-current stimulation to treat stroke patients with aphasia. *Stroke* **41**, 1229–1236.

Barker, A.T., Jalinous, R. & Freeston, I.L. (1985): Non-invasive magnetic stimulation of human motor cortex. *Lancet* **1(8437)**, 1106–1107.

Beck, S., Richardson, S.P., Shamim, E.A., Dang, N., Schubert, M. & Hallett, M. (2008): Short intracortical and surround inhibition are selectively reduced during movement initiation in focal hand dystonia. *J. Neurosci.* **28**, 10363–10369.

Bindman, L.J., Lippold, O.C. & Redfearn, J.W. (1962): Long-lasting changes in the level of the electrical activity of the cerebral cortex produced by polarizing currents. *Nature* **196**, 584–585.

Cantello, R., Tarletti, R. & Civardi, C. (2002): Transcranial magnetic stimulation and Parkinson's disease. *Brain Res. Rev.* **38**, 309–327.

Caramia, M.D., Desiato, M.T., Cicinelli, P., Iani, C. & Rossini, P.M. (1993): Latency jump of 'relaxed' versus 'contracted' motor evoked potentials as a marker of cortico-spinal maturation. *Electroencephalogr. Clin. Neurophysiol.* **89**, 61–66.

Chang, W.H., Kim, Y.H., Bang, O.Y., Kim, S.T., Park, Y.H. & Lee, P.K. (2010): Long-term effects of rTMS on motor recovery in patients after subacute stroke. *J. Rehabil. Med.* **42**, 758–764.

Creutzfeld, O.D., Fromm, G.H. & Kapp, H. (1962): Influence of transcortical dc-currents on cortical neuronal activity. *Exp. Neurol.* **5**, 436–452.

Day, B.L., Dressler, D., Maertens de Noordhout, A., Marsden, C.D., Nakashima, K., *et al.* (1989): Electric and magnetic stimulation of human motor cortex: surface EMG and single motor unit responses. *J. Physiol.* **412**, 449–473.

Di Lazzaro, V., Oliviero, A., Profice, P., Saturno, E., Pilato, F., Insola, A., *et al.* (1998a): Comparison of descending volleys evoked by transcranial magnetic and electric stimulation in conscious humans. *Electroencephalogr. Clin. Neurophysiol.* **109**, 397–401.

Di Lazzaro, V., Restuccia, D., Oliviero, A., Profice, P., Ferrara, L., Insola, A., *et al.* (1998b): Magnetic transcranial stimulation at intensities below active motor threshold activates intracortical inhibitory circuits. *Exp. Brain Res.* **119**, 265–268.

Di Lazzaro, V., Rothwell, J.C., Oliviero, A., Profice, P., Insola, A., Mazzone, P. & Tonali, P. (1999a): Intracortical origin of the short latency facilitation produced by pairs of threshold magnetic stimuli applied to human motor cortex. *Exp. Brain Res.* **129**, 494–499.

Di Lazzaro, V., Oliviero, A., Profice, P., Ferrara, L., Saturno, E., Pilato, F. & Tonali, P. (1999b): The diagnostic value of motor evoked potentials. *Clin. Neurophysiol.* **110**, 1297–1307.

Di Lazzaro, V., Oliviero, A., Meglio, M., Cioni, B., Tamburrini, G., Tonali, P. & Rothwell, J.C. (2000): Direct demonstration of the effect of lorazepam on the excitability of the human motor cortex. *Clin. Neurophysiol.* **111**, 794–799.

Di Lazzaro, V., Oliviero, A., Tonali, P.A., Marra, C., Daniele, A., Profice, P., *et al.* (2002a): Noninvasive in vivo assessment of cholinergic cortical circuits in AD using transcranial magnetic stimulation. *Neurology* **59**, 392–397.

Di Lazzaro, V., Oliviero, A., Mazzone, P., Pilato, F., Saturno, E., Dileone, M., et al. (2002b): Short-term reduction of intracortical inhibition in the human motor cortex induced by repetitive transcranial magnetic stimulation. *Exp. Brain Res.* **147**, 108–113.

Di Lazzaro, V., Oliviero, A., Pilato, F., Saturno, E., Dileone, M., Mazzone, P., et al. (2004a): The physiological basis of transcranial motor cortex stimulation in conscious humans. *Clin. Neurophysiol.* **115**, 255–266.

Di Lazzaro, V., Pilato, F., Oliviero, A., Saturno, E., Dileone, M. & Tonali, P.A. (2004b): Role of motor evoked potentials in diagnosis of cauda equina and lumbosacral cord lesions. *Neurology* **63**, 2266–2271.

Di Lazzaro, V., Pilato, F., Dileone, M., Saturno, E., Oliviero, A., Marra, C., et al. (2006): In vivo cholinergic circuit evaluation in frontotemporal and Alzheimer dementias. *Neurology* **66**, 1111–1113.

Di Lazzaro, V., Pilato, F., Dileone, M., Saturno, E., Profice, P., Marra, C., et al. (2007): Functional evaluation of cerebral cortex in dementia with Lewy bodies. *Neuroimage* **37**, 422–429.

Di Lazzaro, V., Pilato, F., Dileone, M., Profice, P., Marra, C., Ranieri, F., et al. (2008): In vivo functional evaluation of central cholinergic circuits in vascular dementia. *Clin. Neurophysiol.* **119**, 2494–2500.

Dileone, M., Profice, P., Pilato, F., Alfieri, P., Cesarini, L., Mercuri, E., et al. (2010): Enhanced human brain associative plasticity in Costello syndrome. *J. Physiol.* **588**, 3445–3456.

Edwards, M.J., Huang, Y.Z., Mir, P., Rothwell, J.C. & Bhatia, K.P. (2006): Abnormalities in motor cortical plasticity differentiate manifesting and nonmanifesting DYT1 carriers. *Mov. Disord.* **21**, 2181–2186.

Emara, T.H., Moustafa, R.R., Elnahas, N.M., Elganzoury, A.M., Abdo, T.A., Mohamed, S.A. & Eletribi, M.A. (2010): Repetitive transcranial magnetic stimulation at 1 Hz and 5 Hz produces sustained improvement in motor function and disability after ischaemic stroke. *Eur. J. Neurol.* **17**, 1203–1209.

Fitzgerald, P.B., Fountain, S. & Daskalakis, Z.J. (2006): A comprehensive review of the effects of rTMS on motor cortical excitability and inhibition. *Clin. Neurophysiol.* **117**, 2584–2596.

Fregni, F. & Pascual-Leone, A. (2007): Technology insight: noninvasive brain stimulation in neurology-perspectives on the therapeutic potential of rTMS and tDCS. *Nat. Clin. Pract. Neurol.* **3**, 383–393.

Garvey, M.A. & Mall, V. (2008): Transcranial magnetic stimulation in children. *Clin. Neurophysiol.* **119**, 973–984.

Garvey, M.A., Ziemann, U., Bartko, J.J., Denckla, M.B., Barker, C.A. & Wassermann, E.M. (2003): Cortical correlates of neuromotor development in healthy children. *Clin. Neurophysiol.* **114**, 1662–1670.

Gilio, F., Suppa, A., Bologna, M., Lorenzano, C., Fabbrini, G. & Berardelli, A. (2007): Short-term cortical plasticity in patients with dystonia: a study with repetitive transcranial magnetic stimulation. *Mov. Disord.* **22**, 1436–1443.

Heinen, F., Glocker, F.X., Fietzek, U., Meyer, B.U., Lücking, C.H. & Korinthenberg, R. (1998): Absence of transcallosal inhibition following focal magnetic stimulation in preschool children. *Ann. Neurol.* **43**, 608–612.

Hoogendam, J.M., Ramakers, G.M. & Di Lazzaro, V. (2010): Physiology of repetitive transcranial magnetic stimulation of the human brain. *Brain Stimul.* **3**, 95–118.

Huang, Y.Z., Edwards, M.J., Rounis, E., Bhatia, K.P. & Rothwell, J.C. (2005): Theta burst stimulation of the human motor cortex. *Neuron* **45**, 201–206.

Huang, Y.Z., Rothwell, J.C., Lu, C.S., Wang, J. & Chen, R.S. (2010): Restoration of motor inhibition through an abnormal premotor-motor connection in dystonia. *Mov. Disord.* **25**, 689–696.

Hummel, F.C. & Cohen, L.G. (2006): Non-invasive brain stimulation: a new strategy to improve neurorehabilitation after stroke? *Lancet Neurol.* **5**, 708–712.

Khedr, E.M., Ahmed, M.A., Fathy, N. & Rothwell, J.C. (2005): Therapeutic trial of repetitive transcranial magnetic stimulation after acute ischaemic stroke. *Neurology* **65**, 466–468.

Kirton, A., Chen, R., Friefeld, S., Gunraj, C., Pontigon, A.M. & Deveber, G. (2008): Contralesional repetitive transcranial magnetic stimulation for chronic hemiparesis in subcortical paediatric stroke: a randomised trial. *Lancet Neurol.* **7**, 507–513.

Kujirai, T., Caramia, M.D., Rothwell, J.C., Day, B.L., Thompson, P.D., Ferbert, A., et al. (1993): Corticocortical inhibition in human motor cortex. *J. Physiol.* **471**, 501–519.

Maegaki, Y., Maeoka, Y., Ishii, S., Eda, I., Ohtagaki, A., Kitahara, T., et al. (1999): Central motor reorganization in cerebral palsy patients with bilateral cerebral lesions. *Pediatr. Res.* **45**, 559–567.

Mall, V., Berweck, S., Fietzek, U.M., Glocker, F.X., Oberhuber, U., Walther, M., et al. (2004): Low level of intracortical inhibition in children shown by transcranial magnetic stimulation. *Neuropediatrics* **35**, 120–125.

Merton, P.A. & Morton, H.B. (1980): Stimulation of the cerebral cortex in the intact human subject. *Nature* **285**, 227.

Mhalla, A., de Andrade, D.C., Baudic, S., Perrot, S. & Bouhassira, D. (2010): Alteration of cortical excitability in patients with fibromyalgia. *Pain* **149**, 495–500.

Mylius, V., Gerstner, A., Peters, M., Prokisch, H., Leonhardt, A., Hellwig, D. & Rosenow, F. (2009): Low-frequency rTMS of the premotor cortex reduces complex movement patterns in a patient with pantothenate kinase-associated neurodegenerative disease (PKAN). *Neurophysiol. Clin.* **39,** 27–30.

Nitsche, M.A. & Paulus, W. (2000): Excitability changes induced in the human motor cortex by weak transcranial direct current stimulation. *J. Physiol.* **527,** 633–639.

Nitsche, M.A., Cohen, L.G., Wassermann, E.M., Priori, A., Lang, N., Antal, A., *et al.* (2008): Transcranial direct current stimulation: state of the art 2008. *Brain Stimul.* 206–223.

Pilato, F., Dileone, M., Capone, F., Profice, P., Caulo, M., Battaglia, D., *et al.* (2009): Unaffected motor cortex remodeling after hemispherectomy in an epileptic cerebral palsy patient. A TMS and fMRI study. *Epilepsy Res.* **85,** 243–251.

Priori, A., Berardelli, A., Rona, S., Accornero, N. & Manfredi, M. (1998): Polarization of the human motor cortex through the scalp. *Neuroreport* **9,** 2257–2260.

Purpura, D.P. & McMurtry, J.G. (1965): Intracellular activities and evoked potential changes during polarization of motor cortex. *J. Neurophysiol.* **28,** 166–185.

Quartarone, A., Bagnato, S., Rizzo, V., Siebner, H.R., Dattola, V., Scalfari, A., *et al.* (2003): Abnormal associative plasticity of the human motor cortex in writer's cramp. *Brain* **126,** 2586–2596.

Quartarone, A., Siebner, H.R. & Rothwell, J.C. (2006): Task-specific hand dystonia: can too much plasticity be bad for you? *Trends Neurosci.* **29,** 192–199.

Siebner, H.R., Tormos, J.M., Ceballos-Baumann, A.O., Auer, C., Catala, M.D., Conrad, B. & Pascual-Leone, A. (1999): Low-frequency repetitive transcranial magnetic stimulation of the motor cortex in writer's cramp. *Neurology* **52,** 529–537.

Stefan, K., Kunesch, E., Cohen, L.G., Benecke, R. & Classen, J. (2000): Induction of plasticity in the human motor cortex by paired associative stimulation. *Brain* **123,** 572–584.

Terzuolo, C.A. & Bullock, T.H. (1956): Measurement of imposed voltage gradient adequate to modulate neuronal firing. *Proc. Natl. Acad. Sci. USA* **42,** 687–694.

Tokimura, H., Ridding, M.C., Tokimura, Y., Amassian, V.E. & Rothwell, J.C. (1996): Short latency facilitation between pairs of threshold magnetic stimuli applied to human motor cortex. *Electroencephalogr. Clin. Neurophysiol.* **101,** 263–272.

Tokimura, H., Di Lazzaro, V., Tokimura, Y., Oliviero, A., Profice, P., Insola, A., *et al.* (2000): Short latency inhibition of human hand motor cortex by somatosensory input from the hand. *J. Physiol.* **523,** 503–513.

Trompetto, C., Bove, M., Marinelli, L., Avanzino, L., Buccolieri, A. & Abbruzzese, G. (2004): Suppression of the transcallosal motor output: a transcranial magnetic stimulation study in healthy subjects. *Exp. Brain Res.* **158,** 133–140.

Vucic, S., Nicholson, G.A. & Kiernan, M.C. (2008): Cortical hyperexcitability may precede the onset of familial amyotrophic lateral sclerosis. *Brain* **131,** 1540–1550.

Walther, M., Berweck, S., Schessl, J., Linder-Lucht, M., Fietzek, U.M., Glocker, F.X., *et al.* (2009): Maturation of inhibitory and excitatory motor cortex pathways in children. *Brain Dev.* **31,** 562–567.

Zaghi, S., Acar, M., Hultgren, B., Boggio, P.S. & Fregni, F. (2010): Noninvasive brain stimulation with low-intensity electrical currents: putative mechanisms of action for direct and alternating current stimulation. *Neuroscientist* **16,** 285–307.

Ziemann, U., Muellbacher, W., Hallett, M. & Cohen, L.G. (2001): Modulation of practice-dependent plasticity in human motor cortex. *Brain* **124,** 1171–1181.

## Chapter 7

# High-density electroencephalography

### Giuliano Avanzini and Ferruccio Panzica

*Fondazione IRCCS Istituto Neurologico C. Besta, via Celoria 11, 20133 Milan, Italy*
avanzini@istituto-besta.it

### Summary

Electroencephalography (EEG) is a first-line investigational method to study brain function, its strength being its optimal time resolution. In order to compensate for its much less satisfactory space resolution, a method based on a larger number of electrodes (high-density EEG) has been developed. Mathematical processing methods of digitally-recorded EEGs are currently applied to high-density EEGs to deal with the very large number of data that are provided by this technique. In this chapter we discuss the interest in high-density EEG for investigating brain function and for clinical diagnosis and we highlight some novel applications that portend its fuller future potential.

### Introduction

Almost a century after Hans Berger's pioneer recordings of electrical activity from the scalp, electroencephalograpy (EEG) continues to provide students of the nervous system with a first-line investigational method. Indeed, neurophysiology has the unique capacity of describing neural activities in real time at a scale of ms, a property that is obviously highly appreciated when dealing with events like neural ones that last from several μsec to 1–2 ms and propagate at a speed as high as 70 m/s. Much less satisfactory than time resolution is EEG space resolution, which has prompted the development of recording systems based on higher number of electrodes (high-density EEG), which further extends and strengthens the value of EEG among the methods for exploring brain functions and dysfunctions.

### Recording techniques

The bioelectrical signals which make up the EEG are nowadays recorded by PC-based equipment connected to specific electronic devices; the electrodes constitute the interface between these two systems. To ensure inter-subject comparability a system of electrode placement must be employed that ensures a constant relationship between the location of the electrodes and the underlying cerebral structures irrespective of the different size of the heads. The most commonly used electrodes are constructed of Ag/AgCl, or of gold-plated silver positioned on the surface of the scalp according to the international 10–20 system (Jasper, 1958), in which the intervals between the electrodes are 10 per cent or 20 per cent the distance between the nasion and the inion (Fig. 1). In standard diagnostic EEG laboratories 21 electrodes are currently employed, but the 10–20 system allows placement of up to 74 electrodes; further extensions up to 345 electrodes (Fig. 2) are made possible, reducing the intervals between the electrodes to 5 per cent of the nasion–inion distance (10–5 system, Oostenveld & Praamstra, 2001). The main technical improvements that made the high-array EEG system practically usable were the realization of pre-cabled EEG caps (Fig. 3) with built-in multiple cable connection with multichannel amplifiers and the development of signal analysis methods that allow the investigators to deal with the large amount of information provided by the system (see below).

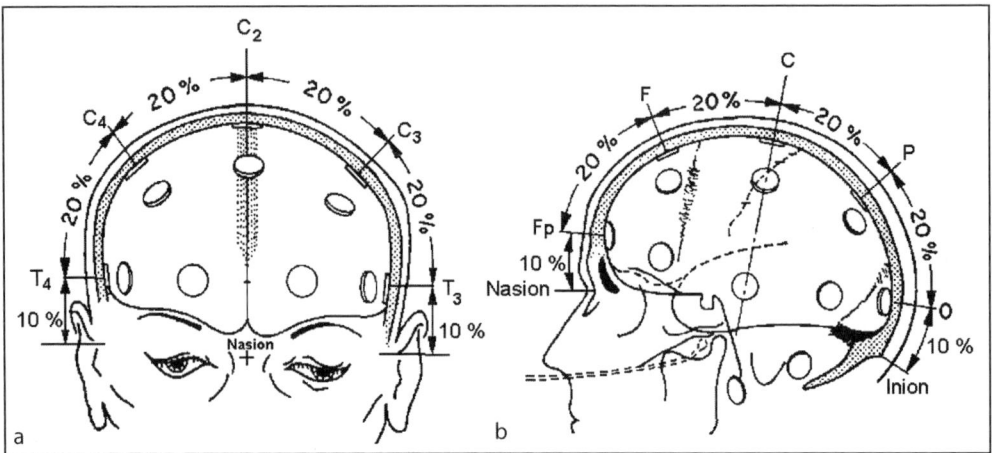

*Fig. 1. Electrode position and labels according to 10–20 system. The electrodes are labelled by capital letters (T for temporal, C for central, Fp for fronto-polar, F for frontal, P parietal, and O for occipital) and numbers (from anterior to posterior, even right, odd left). The midline electrodes are labelled by capital letters plus z ($F_z$, $C_z$, $P_z$. etc.) [From Jasper (1958). Reproduced with permission.]*

Electrical currents related to neuronal activities produce magnetic fields that can be recorded by arrays of superconductors named SQUIDs (superconducting quantum interference devices). The technique of brain magnetic field recording had been standardized under the name of *magnetoencephalography* (MEG) and is now in use in several laboratories. Magnetic fields are less distorted by the resistive properties and inhomogeneities of extracerebral tissues, which confers some advantage of MEG over EEG. Other differences between EEG and MEG signals are that scalp EEG is sensitive to both tangential and radial components of a current source in a spherical volume conductor, whereas MEG detects only its tangential components; thus MEG selectively measures activity in the sulci, while scalp EEG measures activity in the sulci as well as at the top and bottom of the cortical gyri dominated by radial sources. Moreover, the decay of magnetic fields as a function of the distance from the source is more pronounced than for electrical fields, and thus, MEG is more sensitive to superficial cortical activity. Furthermore the magnetic recording is reference-free, whereas the EEG depends on the location of both recording and reference electrodes (Barth & Sutherling, 1986; Cohen & Cuffin, 1983). In general it can be said that MEG can usefully complement EEG, its use being limited by the need of complex and quite expensive facilities (including a shielded room).

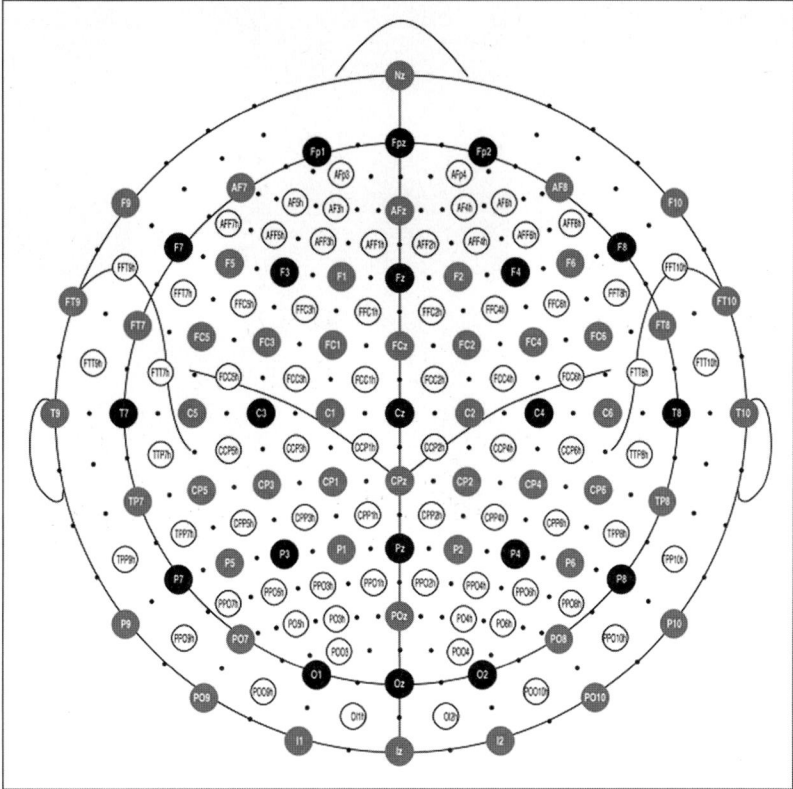

*Fig 2. Electrode positions and labels in the 10–5 International system. Black circles indicate positions of the original 10–20 system; gray circles indicate additional positions (10–10 extension). Positions additional to the 10–10 system are indicated with dots; a selection of additional positions useful for a 128-channel EEG system are indicated with open circles. (From Oostenveld & Praamstra, 2001. Reproduced with permission.)*

## The EEG signal

As soon as he could convince himself that the electrical activity that he recorded from the scalp was indeed generated by the brain, Hans Berger (1929) started to investigate its functional meaning. His efforts, however, did not go far beyond the evidence of a consistent relationship between EEG and states of vigilance. The enormous amount of work devoted to EEG in the following 90 years or so demonstrated that it directly reflects neural mass action, and mainly synchronized postsynaptic potentials of aligned neurons such as pyramidal cells in cortex. Such spatiotemporal synchronization of neural networks results in net polarization of extended brain regions, which may be transient, slow, or oscillatory. The largest EEG potentials are generated by cortical sources which vary in depth and orientation, reflecting the cortical folding. Large populations of cortical neurones can be driven by subcortical structures (namely thalamic nuclei) that may more or less substantially contribute in pacing their discharge.

Some EEG patterns (*e.g.*, spikes) can be directly correlated with the underlying neuronal discharges, and thanks to the development of methods to express proteins in different biological systems, with the molecular mechanisms of neuronal excitability. In particular the expression of mutated channel genes in *Xenopus* oocytes or cultured mammalian cells and the alterations

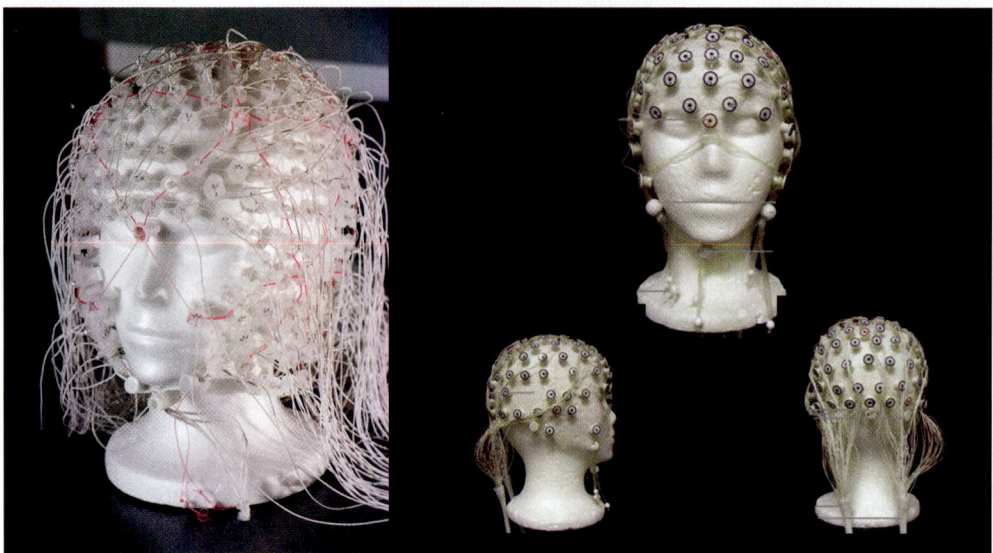

*Fig 3. Commercial precabled caps.*

of transmembrane ionic currents due to dysfunctional, mutated channels have been faithfully characterized. The results of such a combined neurophysiological and biomolecular approach made it possible for the first time to analyze directly the functional effect of channel gene mutations responsible for human genetically determined epilepsies, thus bridging the clinical with the molecular level. In some cases the mutation was found to impair the channel inactivation process, resulting in a prolongation of depolarizing currents (namely, voltage-dependent $Na^+$ currents) that accounted for a hyperexcitable condition. In other cases, the mutation truncates the channel protein, thus abolishing the current. In general the net effect depends on the neuronal population in which the mutation is preferentially expressed: for example, a deletion of $Na^+$ channel alpha 1 subunit that is preferentially expressed in inhibitory neurones results in a hyperexcitable condition in the severe myoclonic epilepsy of infancy, also known as Dravet syndrome (Yu *et al.*, 2006).

In other instances the relationship is more complex.

Although in the past the great EEG value in clinical neurology arose from the empirical observation of the association of some EEG patterns with some brain disorders, we are now witnessing significant advances in the interpretation of the pathophysiologic mechanisms responsible for their generation.

Particular attention has been devoted to the interpretation of the EEG oscillatory activities whose analysis is providing a new approach to neurophysiologic investigation of brain function.

## The EEG rhythms

Electroencephalographic activity is described according to its dominant frequency, amplitude, shape, and distribution over the scalp. Classically the following frequency bands are considered: delta (< 4 Hz), theta (4–7 Hz), alpha (8–12 Hz), beta (13–30 Hz), and gamma (30–70 Hz). These rhythmic activities are largely influenced by thalamic nuclei that are involved in the control of vigilance. In particular, the interaction between inhibitory thalamic reticular neurons and excitatory thalamo-cortical ones are the main ones responsible for the generation of thalamic oscillations. The reciprocal connections between thalamus and cerebral cortex are the anatomo-physiologic bases of thalamo-cortico-thalamic oscillatory systems, which modulate the excitability and responsiveness of cortical neurones with respect to the levels of vigilance (Fig. 4). The effectiveness of an incoming stimulus on a recipient cortical area depends on the frequency and distribution of EEG activities with which it interacts and on the gating effect exerted by thalamic relay nuclei, which may account for the observation that during REM sleep the cerebral cortex is highly active but virtually disconnected from peripheral inputs. Most EEG literature before the 1990s dealt with alpha, theta, and delta bands, but after Singer and Gray's seminal work (1989), many investigations have been devoted to the gamma band and to its correlations with perceptual functions.

To investigate the way by which the information is processed by cerebral cortex, the recording of spontaneous activity has been integrated by event-related potentials (ERPs), which are changes in the ongoing EEG, time-locked (*i.e.*, stimulus- or response-locked) to perceptual, cognitive, or motor processes. They are typically extracted from the ongoing EEG by means of signal averaging. Averaging eliminates not only the spontaneous background EEG, but also those event-related EEG modulations which are not phase-locked as "noise". ERPs consist of characteristic sequences of components or "microstates" (*i.e.*, time segments with a stable topographic distribution of brain electrical activity) that span a continuum between early activity primarily determined by the physical characteristics of the eliciting stimulus (latency range < 250 ms), and later components (latency range > 250 ms) dominated by cognitive rather than physical characteristics of the stimuli (Brandeis & Lehmann, 1986; Picton *et al.*, 2000). The strict time relationship of these evoked responses

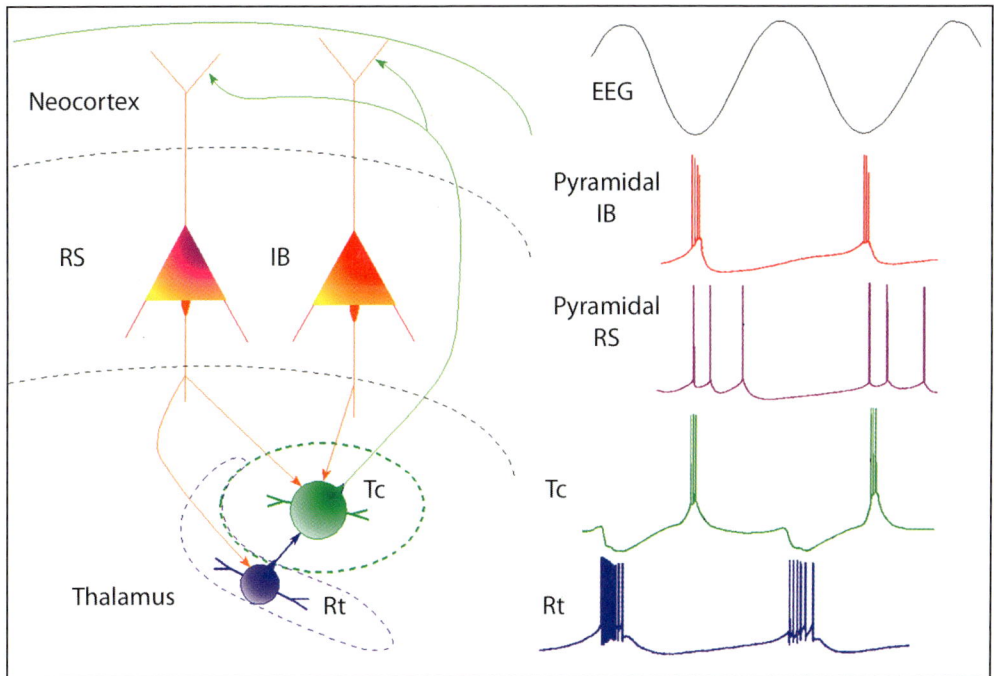

*Fig 4. Thalamic and cortical circuitry involved in the generation of EEG rhythms. RS, regular spiking neocortical pyramidal neurones; IB, intrinsically bursting neocortical pyramidal neurones; Rt, reticular thalamic neurones; Tc, thalamo-cortical thalamic neurones. On the right side of the figure the discharges of the thalamic and cortical neurones are depicted resulting in a cortical EEG rhythm.*

makes it possible to analyze the significance of different components *i.e.*, far-field potentials expressing activity of subcortical relay nuclei *versus* near-field potentials that reflect cortical activation more directly, including the postsynaptic potentials generated in cortical neurons and late, also called cognitive, components that are correlated with higher nervous function. The significance of the different ERP components has been defined to a great extent, however, and their correlation with underlying neuronal activities cannot go beyond the recognition of the involved neuronal networks, while the contribution of different neuronal populations (*e.g.*, excitatory *versus* inhibitory neurones) cannot be resolved with these techniques.

## Signal analysis

The application of mathematical algorithms to analyze the EEG signal allows detection of activities that are otherwise "invisible" by inspective analysis; a typical example of this is the visualization of event-locked activities by the averaging procedure. Moreover, mathematical processing of digitally-recorded EEG is used to quantify the frequency composition (spectral analysis), to analyze or detect specific waveforms, and to define the source of EEG potentials (dipole modeling technique). Signal analysis can be profitably applied to conventional EEG recordings and even more to high-density EEG on account of the very high number of data that can hardly be dealt with by visual inspection. Here we will concentrate on the study of the synchronization of brain oscillations, which provides a new approach to the understanding of the correlation between neuronal activities and the brain's functions (Fig. 5).

Recent studies demonstrated that synchronization of oscillatory brain activity in various frequency bands may be one of the key mechanisms used by the brain to integrate information processed in multiple specialized local brain areas during cognitive tasks or between the central motor system and the periphery. This concept has become known as functional or effective connectivity, the latter aiming at identifying the causal interactions or the direction of information flow between the brain regions studied.

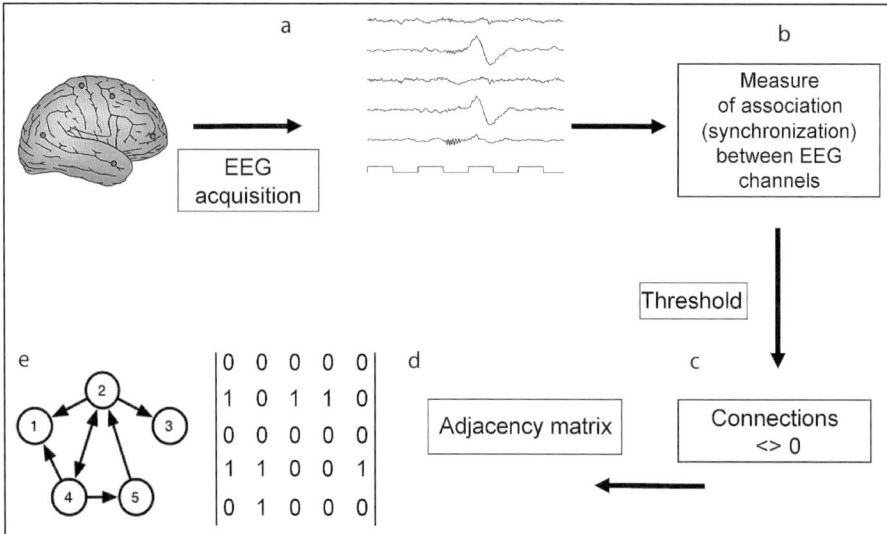

*Fig 5. Flow chart for the estimation of connectivity in a brain network. **a.** High-density EEG recording. **b.** Estimate of a measure of association between EEG channels (nodes). **c.** Generation of an association matrix by determining all pairwise connections between nodes after applying a threshold to each measure. **d.** Production of a binary adjacency matrix. **e.** Calculation of network parameters.*

Integration and segregation of neural activity needs to occur at various spatial and temporal scales, and these scales must be dynamically adjusted depending on the nature of the respective cognitive tasks. Segregation refers to the existence of specialized neurones and brain areas, organized into distinct neuronal populations and grouped together to form segregated cortical areas. The complementary principle, integration, gives rise to the coordinated activation of distributed neuronal populations, thus enabling the emergence of coherent cognitive and behavioural states. The interplay of segregation and integration in brain networks generates information that is simultaneously highly diversified and highly integrated, thus creating patterns of high complexity.

Functional segregation (specialization) and integration have been especially well studied in the visual cortex, which includes several anatomically and physiologically distinct areas, each specialized in the processing of a particular aspect of the visual scene, such as shape, motion, or color. Results of animal experiments indicate that synchronization of neuronal activity in the visual cortex appears to be responsible for the binding of different but related visual features so that a visual pattern can be recognized as a whole (Gray & Singer, 1989, 1995). Moreover, synchronization between areas of the visual and parietal cortex and between areas of the parietal and motor cortex was observed during a visuomotor integration task in the awake cat (Roelfsema *et al.*, 1997). Another piece of evidence is that synchronization of the oscillatory activity in the sensorimotor cortex may serve for the integration and coordination of information underlying motor control. Experimental results demonstrated that in conditions of physiologic excitability, cortical fast activity in the gamma range derives from synchronization of inhibitory GABAergic networks (Bartos *et al.*, 2007; Fries *et al.*, 2007; Whittington & Traub, 2003). According to Fries (2009), the synchronized gamma band activity is originated by excitatory neurones that drive the entire local network, including basket interneurones, which provide shunting inhibition onto each other and onto excitatory neurones. This shunting inhibition will wear off synchronously across the basket cells, which will then fire roughly synchronously. After just a few of these cycles, large numbers of basket cells can be entrained to a rhythm and will impose their rhythmically synchronized inhibition onto the local network's excitatory neurones, which leaves only a short window of opportunity for the excitatory neurones to fire when one bout of inhibition wears off and the next one has not yet arrived. Excitatory inputs are most efficient when they arrive out of phase with the inhibitory barrages, and vice versa. Synchronization can maximize or minimize average gain, dependent on the phase relation (Fig. 6).

Functional neuroimaging studies (fMRI, PET) have indicated that each cognitive process is supported by activated areas extending throughout the brain. The poor temporal resolution (seconds) of the hemodynamic signal is a major shortcoming in the analysis of network timing relations. Studies in human subjects combining EEG and MEG with advanced methods of time-series analysis revealed that neural synchrony is associated with cognitive functions that require large-scale integration of distributed neural activities. For a review, see Singer (1999), Schnitzler & Gross (2005), and Varela *et al.* (2001).

## Clinical applications

The potential of this novel approach based on the study of synchronization (connectivity) of EEG rhythms in different brain areas has so far been demonstrated by few studies dealing with different neurologic and psychiatric disorders. Patients with schizophrenia demonstrate reduced amplitude and synchronization of self-generated, rhythmic activity in several cortical regions [see Ulhaas & Singer (2010) for a review]. Impaired performance in patients with schizophrenia was accompanied by a widespread reduction in the power of gamma-band oscillations in the

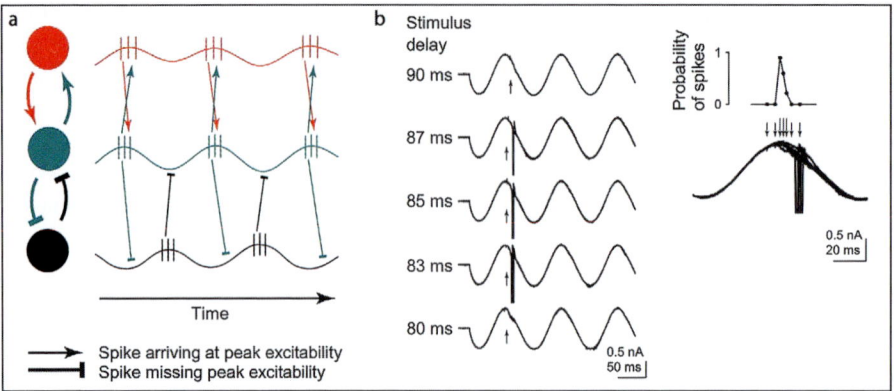

*Fig. 6. Neuronal communication through coherence or phase-locking. **a.** Spikes that arrive at excitability peaks of the receiving neuronal group have pointed arrowheads, whereas those that miss excitability peaks have blunt arrowheads. The red and green neuronal groups undergo coherent excitability oscillations and their communication is effective. **b.** Membrane potentials during injection of sinusoidal current and electrical stimulation of one afferent axon. The timing of the stimulation was varied so that the synaptic input arrived either precisely at its excitability peak or shortly before or after it. (From Fries et al., 2007. Reproduced with permission.)*

right temporal lobe in a time window of 50–300 ms after stimulus onset. These reductions in amplitude are associated with a reduced-phase synchronization of the induced oscillatory activities. Changes in neural oscillations, namely an increase in low-frequency and a reduction in high-frequency activities, have also been demonstrated during rest in schizophrenia: Taken together, these findings suggest that impaired synchronization of beta- and gamma-band oscillations underlies a functional disconnectivity of cortical networks in schizophrenia.

Similar to results obtained in schizophrenia, those in patients with various forms of autism have shown that the dysfunctions in the integration of cognitive mechanisms (Ulhaas & Singer, 2006) may be the result of reduced neural synchronization. Recent fMRI and EEG studies have supported this view (Just *et al.*, 2004).

In the EEGs of patients with remitting-relapsing multiple sclerosis (RRMS) and benign multiple sclerosis (BMS), Vásquez-Marrufo *et al.* (2008) found alterations in the spectral content of different cerebral regions that take place during a visuospatial task. These authors suggest that the observed findings may represent the activation of cortical reorganization processes activated in RRMS patients. Cona *et al.* (2009) analyzed changes in EEG power spectral density and cortical connectivity in healthy and tetraplegic patients during a motor imagery task and found that tetraplegic patients exhibit higher connectivity strength on average, with significant statistical differences in some connections. Jackson and Snyder (2008) reported quantitative EEG to provide a reliable and sensitive biomarker(s) of mild cognitive impairment and early Alzheimer's disease.

Particular attention has been devoted to the localization of epileptic foci on high-density EEG recordings. On 123-channel high-density EEG, Lantz *et al.* (2003), using the EPIFOCUS method (based on a distributed sources model), were able to determine the site of origin of epileptic spikes with an accuracy of 90 per cent. They could also demonstrate that the accuracy is proportional to the number of electrodes employed, thus stressing the importance of high-density EEG. The result is certainly interesting, although its significance needs to be evaluated in the clinical context, knowing that the localization of interictal spikes does not necessarily coincide with the site of origin of the ictal discharge. Further investigations of this technique will tell us whether it is possible to categorize different types of interictal spikes and to define their clinical significance.

## Combination of EEG with other investigation techniques

Polygraphic recordings including EEGs and EMGs are currently used to analyze the relationship between motor phenomena (namely myoclonus) and EEG with the help of some signal analysis techniques (*e.g.*, back averaging). In recent years coherence analysis has been profitably applied to EEG–EMG polygraphic recordings and has provided some interesting information on physiology and pathophysiology of the motor system. Panzica *et al.* (2010) studied EEG–EMG coherence in different progressive myoclonus epilepsy (PME) syndromes with rhythmic myoclonic jerks by means of a time-varying bivariate autoregressive (TVAR) parametric model. Fig. 7 from this study shows a significant EEG–EMG coherence in the beta and gamma bands remaining consistent throughout the movement in a case of sialidosis. Interestingly the method revealed differences in time-frequency spectral profiles between patients with sialidoses and those with Unverricht–Lundborg disease which could be due to different pathophysiologic mechanisms underlying myoclonus. High-density EEG can significantly improve the topographic definition of brain activities related to physiologic and pathophysiologic motor activities.

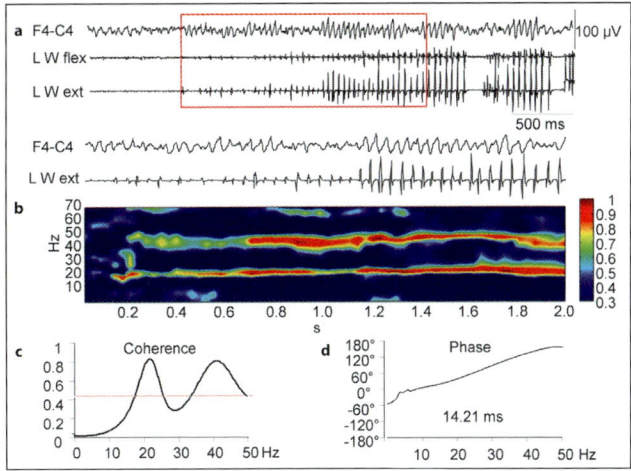

*Fig. 7. Time-varying autoregressive model analysis of a movement-activated myoclonus (**a**) in a patient with sialidosis. Note in the coherence spectrum (**b**) the presence of significant EEG–EMG coherence in the beta and gamma bands, remaining consistent throughout the movement. Panels **c** and **d** display the mean coherence and phase spectra. (From Panzica et al., 2010. Reproduced with permission.)*

Another interesting development is the combination of EEG and functional imaging. This has been made possible as soon as a technique of EEG recording within an MRI machine became available. The EEG-fMRI combination joins the advantage of MRI spatial resolution with EEG time resolution, and the results can be significantly improved by the use of high-density EEG, which makes the spatial definition of the two signals more comparable.

## Conclusions

From the above-reported information it is clear the interest in high-density EEG is not only related to the improvement of spatial resolution, which it provides with respect to conventional EEG, but also to the related advanced techniques of signal analysis. On the one hand, high-density EEG highlights the potential of some types of signal analysis that are optimally applied to it. On the other hand, it significantly contributes to promoting the development of a more sophisticated technique of signal analysis. The results show some novel applications of EEG to the study of brain function and dysfunction that will reveal a fuller potential in the years to come.

## References

Barth, D.S., Sutherling, W.W. & Beatty, J. (1986): Intracellular currents of interictal penicillin spikes: evidence from neuromagnetic mapping. *Brain Res.* **368,** 36–48.

Bartos, M., Vida, I. & Jonas, P. (2007): Synaptic mechanisms of synchronized gamma oscillations in inhibitory interneuron networks. *Nat. Rev. Neurosci.* **8,** 45–56.

Berger, H. (1929): Über das Elektrenkephalogramm des Menschen. *Arch. Psychiatr. Nervenkrank.* **87,** 527–580.

Brandeis, D. & Lehmann, D. (1986): Event-related potentials of the brain and cognitive processes: approaches and applications. *Neuropsychologia* **24,** 151–168.

Cohen, D. & Cuffin, B.N. (1983): Demonstration of useful differences between the magnetoencephalogram and electroencephalogram. *Electroencephalogr. Clin. Neurophysiol.* **56,** 38–51.

Cona, F., Zavaglia, M., Astolfi, L., Babiloni, F. & Ursino M. (2009): Changes in EEG power spectral density and cortical connectivity in healthy and tetraplegic patients during a motor imagery task. *Comput. Intell. Neurosci.* 2009, article ID 279515, 1–12.

Fries, P. (2009): Neuronal gamma-band synchronization as a fundamental process in cortical computation. *Annu. Rev. Neurosci.* **32,** 209–224.

Fries, P., Nikolič, D. & Singer, W. (2007): The gamma cycle. *Trends Neurosci.* **30,** 309–316.

Gray, C.M. & Singer, W. (1989): Stimulus-specific neuronal oscillations in the cat visual cortex. *Proc. Natl. Acad. Sci. USA* **86,** 1698–1702.

Jackson, C. & Snyder, P. (2008): Electroencephalography and event-related potentials as biomarkers of mild cognitive impairment and mild Alzheimer's disease. *Alzheimers Dement.* **4** (Suppl. 1), S137–143.

Jasper, H.H. (1958): The ten twenty electrode system of the International Federation. *Electroenceph. Clin. Neurophysiol.* **10,** 371–375.

Just, M.A., Cherkassky, V.L., Keller, T.A. & Minshew, N.J. (2004): Cortical activation and synchronization during sentence comprehension in high-functioning autism: evidence of underconnectivity. *Brain* **127,** 1811–1821.

Lantz, G., Spinelli, L., Seeck, M., de Peralta Menendez, R.G., Sottas, C.C. & Michel, C.M. (2003): Propagation of interictal epileptiform activity can lead to erroneous source localizations: a 128-channel EEG mapping study. *J. Clin. Neurophysiol.* **20,** 311–319.

Oostenveld, R. & Praamstra, P. (2001): The five per cent electrode system for high-resolution EEG and ERP measurements. *Clin. Neurophysiol.* **112,** 713–719.

Panzica, F., Varotto, G., Canafoglia, L., Rossi-Sebastiano, D., Visani, E. & Franceschetti, S. (2010): EEG-EMG coherence estimated using time-varying autoregressive models in movement-activated myoclonus in patients with progressive myoclonic epilepsies. 32$^{nd}$ Annual International Conference of the IEEE EMBS, Buenos Aires, Argentina, August 31-September 4: 1642–1645.

Picton, T.W., Bentin, S., Berg, P., Donchin, E., Hillyard, S.A., Johnson, R., Jr., et al. (2000): Guidelines for using human event-related potentials to study cognition: recording standards and publication criteria. *Psychophysiology* **37,** 127–152.

Roelfsema, P.R., Engel, A.K., Konig, P. & Singer, W. (1997): Visuomotor integration is associated with zero time-lag synchronization among cortical areas. *Nature* **385,** 157–161.

Schnitzler, A. & Gross, J. (2005): Normal and pathological oscillatory communication in the brain. *Nat. Rev. Neurosci.* **6,** 285–296.

Singer, W. (1999): Neuronal synchrony: a versatile code of the definition of relations? *Neuron* **24,** 49–65.

Singer, W. & Gray, C.M. (1995): Visual feature integration and the temporal correlation hypothesis. *Annu. Rev. Neurosci.* **18,** 555–586.

Ulhaas, P.J. & Singer, W. (2006): Neural synchrony in brain disorders: relevance for cognitive dysfunctions and pathophysiology. *Neuron* **52,** 155–168.

Ulhaas, P.J. & Singer, W. (2010): Abnormal neural oscillations and synchrony in schizophrenia. *Nat. Rev. Neurosci.* **11,** 100–113.

Varela, F., Lachaux, J.P., Rodriguez, E. & Martinerie, J. (2001): The brainweb: phase synchronization and large-scale integration. *Nat. Rev. Neurosci.* **2,** 229–239.

Vázquez-Marrufo, M., González-Rosa, J.J., Vaquero, E., Duque, P., Escera, C., Borges, M., et al. (2008): Abnormal ERPs and high frequency bands power in multiple sclerosis. *Int. J. Neurosci.* **118,** 27–38.

Whittington, M.A. & Traub, R.D. (2003): Interneuron diversity series: inhibitory interneurons and network oscillations in vitro. *Trends Neurosci.* **26,** 676–682.

Yu, F.H., Mantegazza, M., Westenbroek, R.E., Robbins, C.A., Kalume, F., Burton, K.A. & Spain, W.J. (2006): Reduced sodium current in GABAergic interneurons in a mouse model of severe myoclonic epilepsy in infancy. *Nature Neurosci.* **9,** 1142–1149.

## Chapter 8

# Diagnosis of auditory processing disorders

**Elisabetta Genovese, Mariavittoria Vallarino, Maria Consolazione Guarnaccia, and Daniele Monzani**

*Department of Head and Neck, Audiology and Phoniatric Service,*
*University of Modena and Reggio Emilia, largo del Pozzo 71, 41124 Modena, Italy*
elisabetta.genovese@unimore.it

### Summary

Auditory processing disorder (APD) is characterized by the presence of listening difficulties despite a normal audiogram. APD is becoming ever more widely diagnosed in children, although the definition, diagnosis, and aetiology are controverted. This paper deals with the current literature on definition and diagnosis of APD or central auditory processing disorder (CAPD). Because APD is one of the more difficult information-processing disorders to detect and diagnose, it may sometimes be misdiagnosed as ADD/ADHD, Asperger syndrome, and other forms of autism, but it may also be a comorbid aspect of those conditions (Moore, 2006). Interest in diagnosis and management of CAPD spans more than a half-century. Myklebust (1954) stressed the importance of clinically evaluating central auditory function, especially in children affected by communicative disorders. Tests used today to diagnose CAPD have roots in this early work, such as interaural intensity difference training and interhemispheric transfer training). CAPD is an auditory deficit; therefore, the audiologist is the professional who diagnoses CAPD (ASHA, 2005a, 2005b). Although efforts continue to develop more sensitive behavioural tests for the assessment of central auditory function, electrophysiologic, electroacoustic, and neuroimaging procedures may soon transform clinical auditory processing test batteries (see, *e.g.*, the work of Estes *et al.*, 2008). In our clinic, all participants with auditory difficulties are tested with a specific protocol, including audiologic evaluation with audiometry threshold, speech audiometry, and tympanometry. In a second step the patient is tested for his or her ability to understand speech with and without noise.

### Introduction

Auditory processing disorder (APD), also referred to as central auditory processing disorder (CAPD), represents a not-well-defined pathologic entity. Although it does feature in mainstream diagnostic classification such as that of the DSM-IV or ICD-10, APD is becoming more and more a clinical dilemma for professionals in the audiology and developmental sciences.

Hearing impairments arising from central nervous system disorders may have negative consequences for children who are not adequately diagnosed; however, diagnostic and management strategies for these 'central' hearing impairments in childhood are rarely implemented in routine audiologic examinations. These auditory defects have been generally termed 'auditory processing disorders'. A rough prevalence estimate for auditory processing disorders (APDs) in childhood is 7 per cent. Despite the frequency of the problem, a systematic approach to the diagnosis and rehabilitation of APD in children has only started emerging over the past 30 years as a result of developments in the basic sciences; emphasis has shifted from identification of the *lesion* that causes the disorder to identification of the impaired individual's *difficulties* and his or her appropriate rehabilitation.

## Review of the topic

ADP has been defined in a number of ways and refers to how the central nervous system uses auditory information and is not the result of other high-order cognitive, language, or related disorders. ASHA (2005a, 2005b) describes it as an inability to attend to, discriminate, or understand speech under less than optimal conditions, even though peripheral hearing and intelligence are within normal limits; this disability is more marked when listening to distorted speech, in noise, or in other environments with acoustic interference.

Chermak and Musiek (1997) noted that cases of APD with an obvious neurologic aetiology are in the minority (5 per cent). The concept of 'neurodevelopmental disorder' is usually invoked, but its aetiology is not clear, and there is little evidence for the role of any particular risk factor (Dawes *et al.*, 2008). Inherited factors and/or obstetric complications may relate to auditory processing problems, whereas auditory deprivation due to conductive hearing loss (*i.e.*, recurrent otitis media with effusion) has been suggested to underlie only a maturational delay (Chermak *et al.*, 2001). Musiek *et al.* (2005) reported that a genetic determinant was suspected for some children with APD of 'neurodevelopmental origin', the most part of whom have family with histories of learning disabilities. However, Musiek *et al.* (2005) did not distinguish between learning problems such as specific language impairment (SLI), for which there is good evidence for heritability (Bishop, 2006), and more specific auditory problems.

The American Speech-Language Hearing Association (ASHA) published 'Central Auditory Processing Disorders' in January 2005 as an update of the 'Central Auditory Processing: Current Status of Research and Implications for Clinical Practice' (ASHA, 1996) and of the UK's Medical Research Council's Institute of Hearing Research's Auditory Processing Disorder (APD) pamphlet (2004).

The diagnosis of an APD remains a clinical challenge. Poor performance on APD tests does not provide sufficient evidence of an APD. The assessment should enable the clinician to outline the cause of a listening problem and to distinguish auditory problems from language learning or attention deficits which may present in a similar way. A possible confounding factor in the diagnosis of APD must be identified in middle-ear dysfunction, associated with hearing loss (Zumach *et al.*, 2009), in the cross-modal sources such as attention (Sussman & Steinschneider, 2009), the developmental factors (Geva *et al.*, 2008), and the language-learning problems (Shapiro *et al.*, 2009). A better understanding of the consequences of APD and its implications for school performance would provide a basis for selecting the appropriate remedial action that may be needed in each case.

Patients with APD may exhibit a variety of listening and related complaints. For example, they may have difficulties in understanding speech in noisy environments, in following directions, and in discriminating (or telling the difference between) similar-sounding speech sounds. Sometimes they may behave as if a hearing loss is present, often asking for repetition or clarification. In school, children with APD may have difficulties with spelling, reading, and understanding information presented verbally in the classroom (Bishop & McArthur, 2005). However, it is critical to understand that the same symptoms may be apparent in children who do not exhibit APD (Chermak *et al.*, 2007; Musiek *et al.*, 2005). Therefore, we should always keep in mind that not all language and learning problems are due to APD, and all cases of APD do not lead to language and learning problems. APD cannot be diagnosed from a symptoms checklist. No matter how many symptoms of APD a child may have, only careful and accurate diagnostics can determine the underlying cause.

APD refers to how the central nervous system (CNS) processes auditory information. However, the CNS is vast and is also responsible for functions such as memory, attention, and language, among other things. To avoid confusing APD with other disorders that can affect a person's ability to attend, understand, and remember, it is important to emphasize that APD is an auditory deficit that is not the result of other higher-order cognitive, language, or related disorder (King *et al.*, 2002). There are many disorders that can affect a person's ability to understand auditory information. For example, individuals with attention deficit/hyperactivity disorder (ADHD) may well be poor listeners and have difficulty understanding or remembering verbal information (Chermak *et al.*, 2002); however, their actual neural processing of auditory input in the CNS is intact. Instead, the attention deficit itself prevents them from accessing or using the auditory information that is coming in. Children with autism may have great difficulty with spoken-language comprehension. However, it is the higher-order, global deficit known as autism that is the cause of their difficulties, not a specific auditory dysfunction. Finally, although the terms *language* and *auditory processing* are sometimes used interchangeably, it is critical to understand that they are not the same thing at all. For many children and adults with these disorders and others – including mental retardation and sensory integration dysfunction – the listening and comprehension difficulties are due to the higher-order, more global or all-encompassing disorder and not to any specific deficit in the neural processing of auditory stimuli per se (McArthur & Bishop, 2004). So far, it is not correct to apply the label APD to these individuals, even if many of their behaviours appear very similar to those associated with APD. In some cases, however, APD may co-exist with ADHD or other disorders. In those cases, only a careful and an accurate diagnosis can assist in disentangling the relative effects of each (ASHA, 2005b).

A multidisciplinary team approach is necessary to fully assess and understand the complexity of the problems exhibited by children with APD. A teacher or educational advisor may identify academic difficulties; a psychologist may evaluate cognitive functioning and behaviour in a variety of different areas; a speech-language therapist may investigate written and oral language, speech, and related capabilities, and so forth. The actual diagnosis of APD must be finally made by an audiologist, and it is important to know that, however valuable the information from the multidisciplinary team is in understanding the child's overall areas of strength and weakness, none of the tools used by these professionals are in themselves valid to diagnose APD.

To diagnose APD, the audiologist must use a series of tests in a sound-treated room. These tests require listeners to attend to a variety of signals and to respond to them via repetition, pushing a button, or communicating in some other way. Other tests that measure the auditory system's physiologic responses to sound may also be administered, (ASHA, 2005). Most of the tests of APD require that a child be at least 7 or 8 years of age because the variability in brain function is so remarkable in younger children that interpretation of the test results may not be possible.

Once a diagnosis of APD is made, the nature of the disorder is determined (Jerger & Musiek, 2000). There are many types of auditory processing deficits and, because each child is an individual, APD may manifest itself in a variety of ways. Therefore, it is necessary to determine the type of auditory deficit a given child exhibits so that individualized management and treatment may be recommended that address the child's specific areas of difficulty (Musiek, 2004).

According to the British Society of Audiology APD Special Interest Group, the MRC Institute of Hearing Research (2004, retrieved 2008) found people with APD with the following characteristics:

– having trouble paying attention to and remembering information presented orally; these persons cope better with visually acquired information;
– possibly having trouble paying attention and remembering information when information is simultaneously presented in multiple modalities;
– having problems carrying out multi-step directions given orally; they need to hear only one direction at a time;
– appearing to have poor listening skills, and needing people to speak slowly;
– needing more time to process information;
– developing a dislike for locations with background noise such as bars, clubs, or other social locations;
– preferring written communication (*e.g.*, text chat);
– showing behavioural problems.

APD can manifest as problems determining the direction of sounds, difficulty perceiving differences between speech sounds and the sequencing of these sounds into meaningful words, confusing similar sounds such as 'hat' with 'bat', 'there' with 'where', etc. Fewer words may be perceived than were actually said, as there can be problems detecting the gaps between words, creating the sense that someone is speaking unfamiliar or nonsense words. Those suffering from APD may have problems relating what has been said with its meaning, despite obvious recognition that a word has been said, as well as repetition of the word. Background noise, such as the sound of a radio, television, or a noisy bar can make it difficult to impossible to understand speech, depending on the severity of the auditory processing disorder. Using a telephone can be problematic for someone with an auditory processing disorder, in comparison with someone with normal auditory processing, because of low-quality audio, poor signal, and intermittent sounds (Cacace & McFarland, 2005). Many who have auditory processing disorder subconsciously develop visual coping strategies, such as lip-reading, reading body language, and eye contact, to compensate for their auditory deficit, but these coping strategies are not available when using a telephone.

Some of the tests used by educational therapists, neuropsychologists, and educational psychologists give at least an indication that a CAPD might be present. These include tests of auditory memory (for sentences, nonsense syllables, or numbers backward), sequencing, tonal pattern recognition or sound blending, and store of general information (which is most often acquired through listening). The most accurate way to differentiate CAPDs from other problems that mimic them, however, is by clinical audiologic tests of central nervous system function. These are most reliable at locating the site of the problem and reducing the effects of language sophistication on the test results.

CAPD is assessed through the use of special tests designed to assess the various auditory functions of the brain. However, before this type of testing begins, it is important that each person being tested receive a routine hearing test.

It is critical that a complete assessment of the peripheral auditory system, including consideration of auditory neuropathy/auditory dys-synchrony (AN/AD), occur prior to administering a central auditory test battery. At a minimum, this would include evaluation of hearing thresholds, immittance measures (tympanometry and acoustic reflexes), and otoacoustic emissions (OAEs) (Rapin & Gravel, 2003). When contradictory findings exist (*e.g.*, present OAEs combined with absent acoustic reflexes or abnormal hearing sensitivity; abnormal acoustic reflexes with normal tympanometry and OAEs), additional follow-up study should be done to rule out AN/AD before proceeding with central auditory testing (ASHA, 2005).

There are numerous auditory tests that the audiologist can use to assess central auditory function. These fall into two major categories: behavioural tests and electrophysiologic tests. The behavioural tests are often broken down into four subcategories, including monaural low-redundancy speech tests, dichotic speech tests, temporal patterning tests, and binaural interaction tests. It should be noted that children being assessed for CAPD will not necessarily be given a test from each of these categories. Rather, the audiologist will select a battery of tests for each child. The selection of tests will depend upon a number of factors, including the age of the child, the specific auditory difficulties the child displays, the child's native language and cognitive status, and so forth. Most children under the age of 7 years are not candidates for this type of diagnostic testing. In addition, central auditory processing assessments may not be appropriate for children with significant developmental delays (*e.g.*, cognitive deficits) (Rosen *et al.*, 2009).

In our clinical practice, for diagnosis we divided the patients into three categories according to age:

1. Young children, generally under 4 years of age and thus not generally able to cooperate because of their age, undergo audiometric assessment of hearing threshold: (*a*) behavioural audiometry adapted to chronological and/or developmental age (Behavioural Observation Audiometry [BOA], Conditioned Reflex Audiometry [COR], and Visual Reinforcement Audiometry [VRA]; (*b*) otoacoustic emissions (SOAE, TOAE, DPOAE) for study of the cochlear integrity and for the differential diagnosis of cochlear and retrocochlear lesions; (*c*) auditory brainstem responses (ABR) for registration of hearing threshold and for differential diagnosis of conductive and sensorineural loss, and amongst the sensorineural ones, between peripheral and central impairments; (*d*) electrocochleography, when a reliable threshold measure by ABR during spontaneous sleep or conscious sedation could not be obtained because of the child's restlessness, an ABR response appeared unreliable as a threshold indicator for wave-latency functions not in accordance with normative data, the presence of important morphologic abnormalities rendered ABR responses unreliable, or suspected severe hearing loss was associated with serious recurring otitis media with effusion or there was evidence of central nervous system pathologies or central maturation delay.

2. Children between 4 and 7 years of age, who are sent to our clinic for language delay or, in specific cases, for phonologic delay. Audiologic assessment is considered necessary to exclude the auditory deficit as the cause of the language problem. Our test battery to find an auditory processing disorder includes audiologic routine testing and the Children's Word Identification Test (TIPI 1), which examines the ability to identify words differing by a single consonant or vowel sound with four possible choices. The test is composed of four equivalent 50-item lists. The child has to identify a word both in a silent situation and under a competitive noise condition (Arslan *et al.*, 1997). The protocol includes bisyllabic, trisyllabic, and sentence recognition and vowel and confusion phonemic matrix identification under quiet and noisy conditions. The competition noise is characterized by a signal with variable frequency administered at 70 dB; the patients were submitted to all subtests under both conditions.

3. During school age (7 years or older) audiologic appraisal is performed in children with learning disabilities or ADHD. Audiometric assessment of hearing threshold is combined with tests suggested from the literature as auditory discrimination tests and auditory temporal processing and patterning tests, dichotic speech tests, monaural low-redundancy speech tests, binaural interaction tests, and electroacoustic and electrophysiologic measures (ASHA, 2005).

## Conclusions

Clinicians and researchers face many fundamental challenges in trying to define CAPD. Despite several decades of research, neither clinicians nor academics can agree upon a single definition of CAPD. The only practical option available to clinicians is to continuously update their working definitions of CAPD by means of an iterative process based on clinically pragmatic approaches to the diagnosis and rehabilitation of CAPD in real subjects (McArthur, 2009). This option is best achieved by following an audiologic assessment with the purpose of a central auditory diagnostic test battery that examines the integrity of the central auditory nervous system, determines the presence of a CAPD, and describes its parameters. In our experience speech perception tests can be used to identify subjects at risk for APD; the identification of two groups of patients (with/without difficulties in noise conditions) can suggest a possible plan of rehabilitation because children with speech performance reduction under noisy conditions can be considered at risk of developing APD according to the data in the literature.

## References

ASHA: American Speech-Language-Hearing Association (1996): Central auditory processing: current status of research and implications for clinical practice. *Am. J. Audiol.* **5,** 41–54.

ASHA: American Speech-Language-Hearing Association (2005a): Central auditory processing disorder [technical report]. Available at <http://www.asha.org/members/deskref-journals/deskref/default>

ASHA: American Speech-Language-Hearing Association (2005b): Central auditory processing disorder: The role of the audiologist [position statement]. Available at <http://www.asha.org/members/deskref-journals/deskref/default>

Arslan, E., Genovese, E., Orzan, E. & Turrini, M. (1997): *Valutazione della percezione verbale nel bambino ipoacusico.* Bari: Ecumenica.

Bishop, D.V. (2006): What causes specific language impairment in children? *Curr. Dir. Psychol. Sci.* **15,** 217–221.

Bishop, D.V.M. & McArthur, G.M. (2005): Individual differences in auditory processing in specific language impairment: a follow-up study using event-related potentials and behavioural thresholds. *Cortex* **41,** 327–341.

Cacace, A.T. & McFarland, D.J. (2005): The importance of modality specificity in diagnosing central auditory processing disorder. *Am. J. Audiol.* **14,** 112–123.

Chermak, G. (2001): Auditory processing disorder: an overview for the clinician. *Hearing J.* **54,** 10–22.

Chermak, G. & Musiek, F. (1997): *Central Auditory Disorders: New Perspectives.* San Diego, CA: Singular Publishing Group.

Chermak, G.D., Tucker, E. & Seikel, J.A. (2002): Behavioral characteristics of auditory processing disorder and attention-deficit hyperactivity disorder: predominantly inattentive type. *J. Am. Acad. Audiol.* **13,** 332–338.

Chermak, G.D., Silva, M.E., Nye, J., Hasbrouck, J. & Musiek, F.E. (2007): An update on professional education and clinical practices in central auditory processing. *J. Am. Acad. Audiol.* **18,** 428–452; quiz, 455.

Dawes P., Bishop, D.V.M, Sirimanna, T. & Bamiou, D.E. (2008): Profile and aetiology of children diagnosed with auditory processing disorder (APD). *Int. J. Pediatr. Otorhinolaryngol.* **72,** 483–489.

Estes, R.I., Jerger, J. & Jacobson, G. (2008): Reversal of hemispheric asymmetry on auditory tasks in children who are poor listeners. *J. Am. Acad. Audiol.* **13,** 59–71.

Geva, R., Eshel, R., Leitner, Y., Fattal-Valevski, A. & Harel, S. (2008): Verbal short-term memory span in children: long-term modality dependent effects of intrauterine growth restriction. *J. Psychol. Psychiatry* **49,** 1321–1330.

Jerger, J. & Musiek, F. (2000): Report of the Consensus Conference in the diagnosis of auditory processing disorders in school-aged children. *J. Am. Acad. Audiol.* **11,** 467–474.

King, C., Warrier, C.M., Hayes, E. & Kraus, N. (2002): Deficits in auditory brainstem encoding of speech sounds in children with learning problems. *Neurosci. Lett.* **319,** 111–115.

McArthur, G.M. (2009): Auditory processing disorders: can they be treated? *Curr. Opin. Neurol.* **22,** 137–143.

McArthur, G.M. & Bishop, D.V.M. (2004): Which people with specific language impairment have auditory processing deficits? *Cogn. Neuropsychol.* **21,** 79–94.

McArthur, G.M. & Bishop, D.V.M. (2005): Speech and non-speech processing in people with specific language impairment: a behavioural and electrophysiological study. *Brain Lang.* **94,** 260–273.

Medical Research Council, Institute of Hearing Research (2004): *Auditory processing disorder (APD)* [pamphlet]. British Society of Audiology APD Special Interest Group.

Moore, D.R. (2006): Auditory processing disorder (APD): Definition, diagnosis, neural basis, and intervention. *Audiol. Med.* **4,** 4–11.

Musiek, F.E. (2004): Hearing and the brain: audiological consequences of neurological disorders [special issue]. *J. Am. Acad. Audiol.* **15(2).**

Musiek, F.E., Bellis, T.J. & Chermak, G.D. (2005): Nonmodularity of the central auditory nervous system: Implications for (central) auditory processing disorder. *Am. J. Audiol.* **14,** 128–138.

Myklebust, H. (1954): *Auditory Disorders in Children: A Manual for Differential Diagnosis.* New York: Grune & Stratton.

Rapin, I. & Gravel, J. (2003): Auditory neuropathy: physiologic and pathologic evidence calls for more diagnostic specificity. *Int. J. Pediat. Otorhinolaryngol.* **67,** 707–728.

Rosen, S., Cohen, M. & Vanniasegaram, I. (2009): Auditory and cognitive abilities of children suspected of auditory processing disorder (APD). *Int. J. Pediat. Otorhinolaryngol.* **106,** 610–612.

Shapiro, L.R., Hurry, J., Masterson, J., Wydell, T.N. & Doctor, E. (2009): Classroom implications of recent research into literacy development: from predictors to assessment. *Dyslexia* **15,** 1–22.

Sussman, E. & Steinschneider, M. (2009): Attention effects on auditory scene analysis in children. *Neuropsychologia* **47,** 771–785.

Vanniasegaram, I., Cohen, M. & Rosen, S. (2004): Evaluation of selected auditory tests in school-aged children suspected of auditory processing disorder (APD). *Ear Hearing* **25,** 586–597.

Wible, B., Nicol, T. & Kraus, N. (2005). Correlation between brainstem and cortical auditory processes in normal and language-impaired children. *Brain* **128,** 417–423.

Zumach, A., Gerrits, E., Chenault, M.N. & Anteunis, L.J.C. (2009): Otitis media and speech-in-noise recognition in school-aged children. *Audiol. Neurootol.* **14,** 121–129.

## Chapter 9

# Muscle MRI: phenotype–genotype correlation

Eugenio Mercuri, Flaviana Bianco, Gessica Vasco and Marika Pane

*Child Neurology Unit, Policlinico Gemelli, Catholic University, largo A. Gemelli 8, 00168 Rome, Italy*
*mercuri@rm.unicatt.it*

### Summary

This paper compares the advantages of muscle MRI over those of its predecessors – ultrasound and computerized tomography. A short explanation of the physics and sequential procedures of MRI is presented and a short protocol proposed that can be used in very young patients. Additionally we report on the use of muscle MRI in differentiating a number of genetically caused neuromuscular disorders and describe the patterns of the muscles' involvement as observed on scans. MRI findings in concert with spectroscopy or additional sequences may also help to clarify the mechanisms underlying muscle-specific changes in individual disorders, and it is hoped that MRIs will prove of value in monitoring changes over time after intervention.

### Introduction

After the introduction of ultrasound scans as a diagnostic tool in neuromuscular disorders in the 1980s, neuromuscular imaging has become more widely available. Consequently, in the last decade several studies have reported the value of neuromuscular imaging as a complement to clinical and neurophysiologic examination to detect muscle involvement in inherited neuromuscular disorders.

Early studies using muscle ultrasound (US) have already suggested that imaging can be used as a screening exam to detect muscular involvement and to guide procedures such as muscle biopsy by selecting relatively spared muscles (Heckmatt *et al.*, 1980, 1982; Zuberi *et al.*, 1999). The advantages of muscle US are that it is a low-cost, noninvasive technique and rather easy to use. However, its use, compared to that of more advanced techniques, such as muscle computer tomography (CT) and magnetic resonance imaging (MRI), is limited as it is not always easy to visualize the involvement of the deeper muscles in severely affected patients who have a marked involvement of the muscles closer to the probe (Heckmatt *et al.*, 1985).

Computerized tomography has also been widely used. Compared to US, CT is not operator-dependent, and allows a better view of deeper muscles in severely compromised patients (Gozzoli *et al.*, 1990). Its use is, however, mainly limited by the use of ionizing radiation.

The advent of muscle MRI has completely replaced the use of CT. Even if the time required to obtain the images is longer, there are several advantages in using MRI compared to US and CT. MRI is not operator-dependent, it does not require ionizing radiation, and allows the use of multiplanar scanning, which is particularly useful for patients with severe limb contractures who are unable to lie in the correct position during the examination. Furthermore, comparative studies using both CT and MRI techniques have shown that MRI has a higher sensitivity than CT for identifying early fatty replacement in muscles (Ozsarlak *et al.*, 2001; Shedel *et al.*, 1992) and provides better anatomic details (Mercuri *et al.*, 2007).

## Physics and protocols of MRI

The principal sources of the MRI signal are fat and water. Abnormalities causing a change in fat or water content result in altered T1 and T2 relaxation times. Healthy muscle has a long T1 relaxation time, whereas fat has a relatively short and water a long T1 relaxation time. T1-weighted (T1W) images are thus very sensitive in detecting fatty deposition in muscle. In the T2-weighted images, healthy muscle has a short relaxation time, whereas fat and water have long relaxation times. Consequently T2-weighted images are very sensitive to fat and water increases and can show abnormalities earlier than the T1 images because of the increased water content resulting from inflammation or increased blood flow (Curiel *et al.*, 2009). Considering that both fat and water are bright on T2-weighted images, fat cannot always be distinguished from oedema using these sequences. Additional sequences, such as short tau inversion recovery (STIR), can identify oedema and water, removing the signal originating from fat.

The use of multiple sequences therefore can also help to provide more accurate information on the mechanisms underlying the changes seen on imaging. More specifically, multiple sequences can help, for example, to quantify the extent of muscle disease and the diffuse or selective involvement, to differentiate active (oedema as increased signal on T2) from chronic (fat replacement as increased signal on T1) disease, and to quantify the gradient of involvement with different intensity of brightness.

A protocol including all these sequences will therefore allow combining information from the individual sequences, but this is not always a feasible option in young children or in those patients with contractures or respiratory problems who cannot spend too much time lying in the scanner. Because of this we have proposed a short protocol that can be used even in patients as young as 4 or 5 years of age (Mercuri *et al.*, 2002a). In this protocol T1W images are obtained in the leg, and the axial plane is selected with respect to the long axis of the body. This involves two sequential scans (one for the hip and thighs and the other for calves). Each scan provides multiple images for each segment. The slices are 5-mm thick and the gap between slices is 20–50 mm, depending on the size of the child. The total time of the exam is less than 30 minutes, and with an appropriate scoring system it become fast and quite easy to identify different signals in different muscles, recognizing a gestalt of overall pattern. This protocol allows changes in T1 to be easily seen, and the protocol has been successfully used in many studies reporting selective patterns of muscle involvement in several neuromuscular disorders.

## Muscle MRI in neuromuscular disorders

A complete review of the value of muscle MRI in individual neuromuscular disorders is beyond the aims of this chapter as comprehensive recent updates on this topic are already available (Mercuri *et al.*, 2005a, 2007). In this chapter we will report how muscle MRI has been used in the last few years as a valuable tool in the differential diagnosis of neuromuscular disorders sharing clinical and pathologic features. Following the identification of an always increasing number of genes, muscle MRI has been increasingly used to help in differential diagnosis.

We have recently reported how MRI can identify consistent patterns in selective muscle involvement in a group of neuromuscular diseases with rigid spine as a prominent feature (Mercuri et al., 2010). This group includes different congenital muscular dystrophies genetically defined, such as rigid spine muscular dystrophy 1 (RSMD1), Bethlem myopathy (BM), Ullrich congenital muscular dystrophy (UCMD), limb girdle muscular dystrophy 2A (LGMD2A), and autosomal dominant Emery–Dreifuss muscular dystrophy variant (EDMD2). Despite a significant clinical overlap, the five forms are related to different genes and have been reported to have disease-specific patterns of muscle involvement.

RSMD1 is a congenital muscular dystrophy, caused by mutations in SEPN1 and characterized by slowly progressive weakness, rigid spine, and early respiratory failure. The typical pattern of muscle involvement in RSMD1 was originally described (Flanigan et al., 2000) in 2000 in four siblings and subsequently confirmed in another six cases from five families (Mercuri et al., 2002b). In RSMD1, at mid-thigh level, muscle imaging shows a selective involvement of the adductors, sartorius, and biceps femoris more markedly involved and rectus femoris and gracilis relatively spared (Fig. 1). In the lower part of the leg, the gastrocnemius is the most involved muscle, followed by extensor digitorum and peroneal. The selectivity in the thigh muscles is more pronounced early in the disease course followed by widespread muscular signal abnormalities in the late stages of the disease.

This pattern is different from those observed in BM and UCMD, two neuromuscular disorders caused by mutations in three genes (COL6A1, COL6A2, or COL6A3) encoding for the three chains of collagen 6. The typical pattern observed in BM is characterized by prevalent and striking involvement of vasti muscle with a concentric involvement and a rim of abnormal signs at the periphery of the muscle and relative sparing of the central area (Fig. 2). Another peculiar finding of BM is also the 'central shadow' sign, a small area of increased signal on T1 or increased echo on US due to the involvement of the central area of the rectus femoris muscle (Mercuri et al., 2002c).

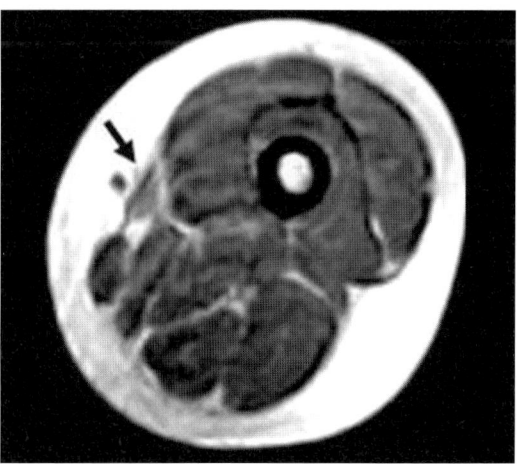

Fig. 1. T1 transverse image of the thigh in a patient with SEPN1 mutations showing the selective involvement of the sartorius muscle.

In UCMD, the more severe form of muscle involvement related to COL6 mutations, there is a diffuse involvement of the thigh muscles with relative sparing of sartorius, gracilis, and adductor longus. As in BM as well as in UCMD there is a pattern of concentric involvement of the vasti lateralis. In contrast the 'central shadow' is less frequent than in BM patients. At calf level, there is a common feature characterized by a rim of peripheral involvement between the soleus and gastrocnemius muscles. Interestingly, despite a more severe impairment shown in UCMD, it is possible to detect this finding also in the overall more diffuse involvement. Although the two patterns are quite distinct there is a significant overlap between the two forms (Mercuri et al., 2005b).

LGMD2A is caused by mutations in CAPN 3, the gene encoding for calpain. The clinical features are variable and it can be difficult to make a diagnosis based on clinical grounds only. MRI has proved to be useful in the differential diagnosis identifying a pattern that is consistent among patients with LGMD2A, but different from that observed in other forms. Muscle MRI shows a predominant posterior thigh involvement with specific impairment of adductor muscles and of the semimembranosus muscle. In patients with the more severe phenotype, there is a similar involvement, but it is associated with more diffuse involvement of the posterior thigh muscles and vasti intermedius and vastus lateralis. At the calf level there is a striking involvement of the medial head of the gastrocnemius muscle compared to the lateral head, which is always relatively spared. The involvement of the gastrocnemius is associated with variable involvement of the soleus muscle (Mercuri et al., 2005c).

The autosomal dominant Emery–Dreifuss muscular dystrophy variant is caused by mutations in LMNA. The features of this form are characterized by slowly progressive muscle weakness and wasting, beginning in muscles of the upper parts of the arms and the lower parts of the legs and progressing to muscles in the shoulders and hips. Contractures involving the elbows, ankles, and neck are very common. In these patients there is a characteristic involvement of the posterior calf muscles that resembles that observed in LGMD2A, but with a different involvement of the thigh muscles (Mercuri et al., 2002d). As in LGMD2A, the medial head of the gastrocnemius is always predominantly involved, whereas the lateral head is relatively spared. This pattern is more obvious in mildly affected patients in whom the other calf muscles are spared or only mildly involved, but it is also recognizable in the patients with more advanced disease. The involvement at thigh level is different, however, from that observed in LGMD2A (Fischer et al., 2005), with a variable involvement, often associated with a predominant involvement of the vasti muscles.

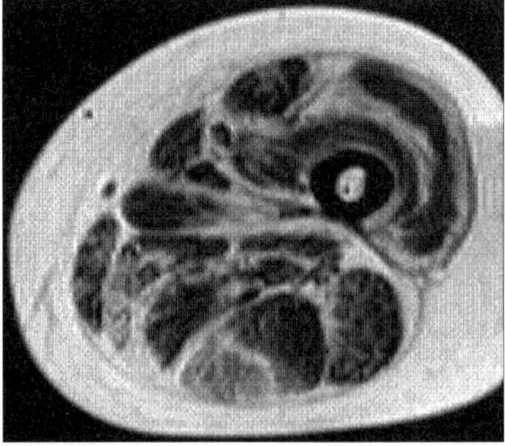

*Fig. 2. T1 transverse image of the thigh in a patient with Bethlem myopathy showing typical changes at the periphery of the vastus lateralis with sparing of the internal part and selective involvement of the central part of the rectus femoris.*

In a recent study (Mercuri *et al.*, 2010), we have assessed how specific these findings are to identify different disorders. The study was performed analyzing muscle MRI scans in 83 patients affected by five genetically distinct muscular dystrophy variants, all associated with spine rigidity, with another control group of 25 patients with other forms of muscular dystrophies to establish the specificity of the patterns found in the study group. The analysis of the scans was performed using a gestalt interpretation, looking at the overall pattern of muscle involvement. In this way, it was possible to define a peculiar pattern in which individual muscles or groups of muscles were specifically spared or involved according to the disease.

The scans were reviewed by examiners who had some expertise in MRI, but were not all radiologists. Each scan was compared with the published examples of the typical patterns observed in patients affected by the five forms of muscular dystrophies with associated spine rigidity.

The scans were classified into four different categories: *typical* if they were similar to the patterns already reported in literature; *consistent* but not strictly typical if the patterns observed were quite similar to those observed, but had additional or missing features; *different* if a pattern could be identified but was different from the five previously reported; or *uninformative* if the changes were absent or minimal, therefore affecting the possibility of assigning any pattern of muscle involvement.

The results of this study showed that the gestalt interpretation of the overall pattern of muscle involvement has a good sensitivity (0.9) and specificity (0.96) in detecting typical changes consistent with those previously reported. In this group, approximately 10 per cent of the scans were uninformative, with only minimal changes that did not allow any pattern recognition. False-negative results represented a relatively low rate and were not related to the age of the patient (five of the eight patients with uninformative scans were in their teens or adults). In the remaining 75 cases, the patterns were classified as 'typical' (67/83) or at least 'consistent' (7/83) of one of the five patterns of the forms of MD associated with spinal rigidity provided as examples. The patterns identified were consistent with the appropriate clinical and genetic diagnosis in 74 of the 75, with only one false-positive result. The specificity of these findings is further increased by the fact that in the control group, all patients had some muscle changes, but in none were the patterns identified similar to those found in our study group.

## Conclusions

These results are just an example of how MRI findings can also help in targeting the genetic investigations. Other techniques such as spectroscopy or additional sequences may help to better elucidate the different mechanisms underlying muscle-specific distribution of changes in individual disorders. Collaborative international work is also in progress to establish the value of muscle MRI as an outcome measure to monitor changes over time after intervention.

## References

Curiel, R.V., Jones, R. & Brindle, K. (2009): Magnetic resonance imaging of the idiopathic inflammatory myopathies: structural and clinical aspects. *Ann. N. Y. Acad. Sci.* **1154,** 101–114.

Fischer, D., Walter, M.C., Kesper, K., Petersen, J.A., Aurino, S., Nigro, V., *et al.* (2005): Diagnostic value of muscle MRI in differentiating LGMD2I from other LGMDs. *J. Neurol.* **252,** 538–547.

Flanigan, K.M., Kerr, L., Bromberg, M.B., Leonard, C., Tsuruda, J., Zhang, P., *et al.* (2000): Congenital muscular dystrophy with rigid spine syndrome: a clinical, pathological, radiological, and genetic study. *Ann Neurol.* **47,**152–161.

Gozzoli, G., Ottolini, A. & Uggetti, C. (1990): La tomografia computerizzata nello studio delle malattie neuromuscolari II. *Riv. Neuroradiol.* **3,** 223–231.

Heckmatt, J.Z. & Dubowitz, V. (1985): Diagnostic advantage of needle muscle biopsy and ultrasound imaging in the detection of focal pathology in a girl with limb girdle dystrophy. *Muscle Nerve* **8,** 705–709.

Heckmatt, J.Z., Dubowitz, V. & Leeman, S. (1980): Detection of pathological change in dystrophic muscle with B-scan ultrasound imaging. *Lancet* **1,** 1389–1390.

Heckmatt, J.Z., Leeman, S. & Dubowitz, V. (1982): Ultrasound imaging in the diagnosis of muscle disease. *J. Pediatr.* **101,** 656–660.

Mercuri, E., Pichiecchio, A., Counsell, S., Allsop, J., Cini, C., Jungbluth, H., *et al.* (2002a): A short protocol for muscle MRI in children with muscular dystrophies. *Eur. J. Paediatr. Neurol.* **6,** 305–307.

Mercuri, E., Talim, B., Moghadaszadeh, B., Petit, N., Brockington, M., Counsell, S., *et al.* (2002b): Clinical and imaging findings in six cases of congenital muscular dystrophy with rigid spine syndrome linked to chromosome 1p (RSMD1). *Neuromuscul Disord.* **12,** 631–638.

Mercuri, E., Cini, C., Counsell, S., Allsop, J., Zolkipli, Z., Jungbluth, H., *et al.* (2002c): Muscle MRI findings in a three-generation family affected by Bethlem myopathy. *Eur. J. Paediatr. Neurol.* **6,** 309–314.

Mercuri, E., Counsell, S., Allsop, J., Jungbluth, H., Kinali, M., Bonne, G., *et al.* (2002d): Selective muscle involvement on magnetic resonance imaging in autosomal dominant Emery-Dreifuss muscular dystrophy. *Neuropediatrics* **33,** 10–14.

Mercuri, E., Jungbluth, H. & Muntoni, F. (2005a): Muscle imaging in clinical practice: diagnostic value of muscle magnetic resonance imaging in inherited neuromuscular disorders. *Curr. Opin. Neurol.* **18,** 526–537.

Mercuri, E., Lampe, A., Allsop, J., Knight, R., Pane, M., Kinali, M., *et al.* (2005b): Muscle MRI in Ullrich congenital muscular dystrophy and Bethlem myopathy. *Neuromuscul. Disord.* **15,** 303–310.

Mercuri, E., Bushby, K., Ricci, E., Birchall, D., Pane, M., Kinali, M., *et al.* (2005c): Muscle MRI findings in patients with limb girdle muscular dystrophy with calpain 3 deficiency (LGMD2A) and early contractures. *Neuromuscul. Disord.* **15,** 164–171.

Mercuri, E., Pichiecchio, A., Allsop, J., Messina, S., Pane, M. & Muntoni, F. (2007): Muscle MRI in inherited neuromuscular disorders: past, present, and future. *J. Magn. Res. Imaging* **25,** 433–440.

Mercuri, E., Clements, E., Offiah, A., Pichiecchio, A., Vasco, G., Bianco, F., *et al.* (2010): Muscle magnetic resonance imaging involvement in muscular dystrophies with rigidity of the spine. *Ann. Neurol.* **67,** 201–208.

Ozsarlak, O., Schepens, E., Parizel, P.M., Van Goethem, J.W., Vanhoenacker, F., De Schepper, A.M. & Martin, J.J. (2001): Hereditary neuromuscular diseases. *Eur. J. Radiol.* **40,** 184–197.

Schedel, H., Reimers, C.D., Nägele, M., Witt, T.N., Pongratz, D.E. & Vogl, T. (1992): Imaging techniques in myotonic dystrophy. A comparative study of ultrasound, computed tomography and magnetic resonance imaging of skeletal muscles. *Eur. J. Radiol.* **15,** 230–238.

Zuberi, S.M., Matta, N., Nawaz, S., Stephenson, J.B., McWilliam, R.C. & Hollman, A. (1999): Muscle ultrasound in the assessment of suspected neuromuscular disease in childhood. *Neuromuscul. Disord.* **9,** 203–207.

## Chapter 10

# Functional MRI in children: clinical applications

### Andrea Zsoter* and Martin Staudt°

*Department of Neuropediatrics and Developmental Medicine,
Experimental Paediatric Neuroimaging, University Children's Hospital,
Hoppe-Seyler-Str.1, 72076 Tübingen, Germany
°Neuropediatric Clinic and Clinic for Neurorehabilitation,
Epilepsy Center for Children and Adolescents,
Schön-Klinik Vogtareuth, Krankenhausstr. 20, 83569 Vogtareuth, Germany
Andrea.Zsoter@med.uni-tuebingen.de
mstaudt@schoen-kliniken.de

### Summary

Functional MRI (fMRI) is a noninvasive tool to localize brain function and is widely used in the field of neuroscience research since the 1990s. In recent years its clinical application has increased in adults as well as in children. This article describes the major indications and methods of clinical fMRI in children and illustrates them with case reports.

Localization of sensorimotor and language functions, sometimes visual functions, are the main domains for clinical fMRI. The tasks which have been developed are child-friendly and can be used even in young children. Presurgical evaluation is the main indication for fMRI, either in children with brain tumours or with refractory epilepsies during the process of planning epilepsy surgery. The results of clinically indicated fMRI have to be part of a set of diagnostic tools. Especially the question of re-organization of the sensorimotor system can often only be answered using the complementary method of transcranial magnetic stimulation (TMS). Verifying or disproving suspected re-organization of sensorimotor or language function can be crucial for counselling patients and parents in the decision-making process in elective epilepsy surgery. Knowing the spatial relationship of functional areas (through fMRI) and tracts (*e.g.*, pyramidal tract) through the technique of diffusion tensor imaging (DTI) has become a helpful tool in paediatric neurosurgery.

### Introduction

Functional MRI (fMRI), a noninvasive method for localization of functional brain regions, has become generally available beginning in the 1990s and is now a widely used tool both in neuroscience research and in clinical investigation. Functional MRI uses the blood oxygen level–dependency (BOLD) effect, the difference of oxygen availability during times of activation and times of rest, which can be visualized by means of the paramagnetic properties of deoxyhemoglobin (Ogawa, 1990). So-called T2* sequences in the echo planar imaging technique (EPI) are used for fMRI [for further details, see the review of Norris (2006)]. Contraindications are the same as for structural MRI of the brain, but, in addition, a greater compliance to perform the tasks is needed.

**Indications and methods**

Even if the main domain of fMRI is neuroscience research, it has now become an important diagnostic tool in clinical evaluation of patients in the last several years. The localization of sensorimotor, language, and sometimes visual functions are the major indications for fMRI in children as part of presurgical evaluation in an effort to treat drug-resistant epilepsies or brain tumours, both in the vicinity of (functional) critical structures. Furthermore, reorganization of any of these functions needs to be evaluated in children with early brain lesions prior to elective surgery.

In younger or psychomotor-handicapped children it is especially important to adapt the fMRI tasks to child-friendly versions. Because head movement is the main problem, the time for one task needs to be shorter than in adults and the task should be interesting in order to attract the child's attention and not too difficult to ensure performance (Wilke, 2003).

Children need to be instructed carefully before undergoing fMRI. Most of the children are somewhat familiar with MRI procedures because they have often had a structural MRI before. But if this was done under sedation or anaesthesia, it is recommended that the child becomes familiarized with the scanner, perhaps by letting the child lie on the bench and by answering his or her questions, possibly one day before the examination is scheduled. All planned tasks need to be explained in detail, and sometimes it is a good idea for the child to 'practice' ahead of time with their parents. In younger children, the examination can be performed more easily if one of the parents is accompanying the child (*e.g.*, holding one hand on the child's leg). Before starting the scan, the examiner should make sure that the child is comfortable in the scanner, because discomfort can result in excessive movements or abruption. In general fMRI in children is performed in a block design of alternating active and control or rest conditions because the signal-to-noise ratio is much better in block- than event-related design (Carter, 2008). In the following chapter indications and techniques of clinical fMRI in children are explained and illustrated with an emphasis on case examples.

**Sensorimotor system**

With fMRI, the somatotopic representation of the motor cortex can be shown noninvasively (Lotze *et al.*, 2000). The major tasks in clinical application are active or passive movement of the hand or toes and sometimes active lip movement.

To perform fMRI in younger, less cooperative, or mentally handicapped children some modifications are necessary (Guzzetta *et al.*, 2007; Staudt *et al.*, 2001). In our setting, children are instructed to squeeze the hand or the index finger of the examiner, which has two advantages compared to the instruction in adults to perform a certain movement (finger opposition or hand movements). First, there is a direct contact between the young patient and the examiner, which allows the examiner to 'feel' the task performance; second, this physical contact reduces fear in anxious patients and therefore helps to facilitate the examination. The scanner protocol itself is also modified. The repetition time between the scan-acquisitions is doubled and this extra time is used to give repetitive instructions to the child (to continue squeezing, to close the eyes again, not to move, *etc.*) or to reassure the child ('you are doing fine'). In order to achieve the same amount of data, but not to prolong one run, each task is done twice and analyzed together (Staudt *et al.*, 2001; Staudt *et al.*, 2004a). If the child cannot perform hand movements without a lot of associated movements, which would lead to excessive movement artefacts, the evaluation can be done with passive movement of the hand (Guzzetta *et al.*, 2007) – with some cautions in interpretation, as shown later.

**Case one** is a 3-year-old boy with therapy-refractory epilepsy due to a suspected focal cortical dysplasia in the precentral gyrus. The boy had no hemiparesis. As part of the presurgical evaluation of treatment options, he was sent for fMRI for localization of the primary sensorimotor area of the hand. After carefully instructing the child, the fMRI was performed in the above-described 'child modus'; instead of squeezing the examiner's finger, the boy squeezed a toy. The child's mother was next to the child in the scanner room and the examination could successfully be done. Fig. 1 shows the activation for active hand movement and displays the relationship between the sensorimotor hand representation and the focal cortical dysplasia. This example shows that clinical fMRI can be performed even in very young children (Staudt *et al.*, 2005).

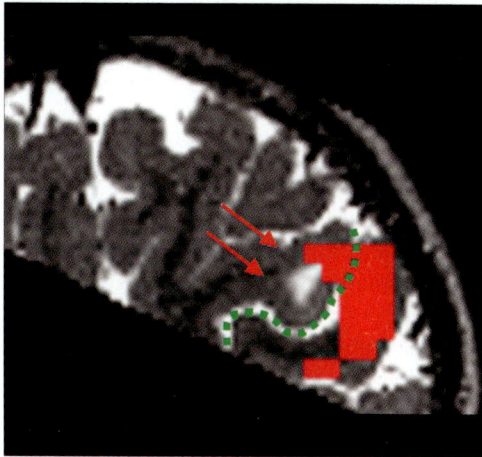

*Fig. 1. Activation after active movement of the hand in the primary sensorimotor area close to the dysplasia (red arrows) in a 3-year-old boy (green dotted line: central sulcus) (fMRI superimposed on T2 high-resolution structural MRI from Prof. Winkler, Stuttgart). (Reprinted with permission from Staudt, 2010).*

**Case two** is a 6-year-old girl with a slowly growing tumour in the right frontal lobe, presenting with focal epilepsy several years ago. The girl had no motor impairment. Prior to planned neurosurgery because of tumour growth, the girl underwent a functional MRI of the hand and a structural MRI with additional diffusion tensor imaging.

The fMRI was done in the 'child modus' and repeated twice, showing a reproduced activation area close to the tumour. The functional data were imported to iPlan 2.6, Brainlab, and fibre tracking was done to visualize the corticospinal motor and spino-thalamo-cortical somatosensory projections (Fig. 2). After exporting the data to the intraoperative neuronavigation system, the neurosurgeons were able to have further visual guidance regarding the close relationship between the tumour and descending corticospinal projections, which led to a complete tumour resection without neurologic deficit.

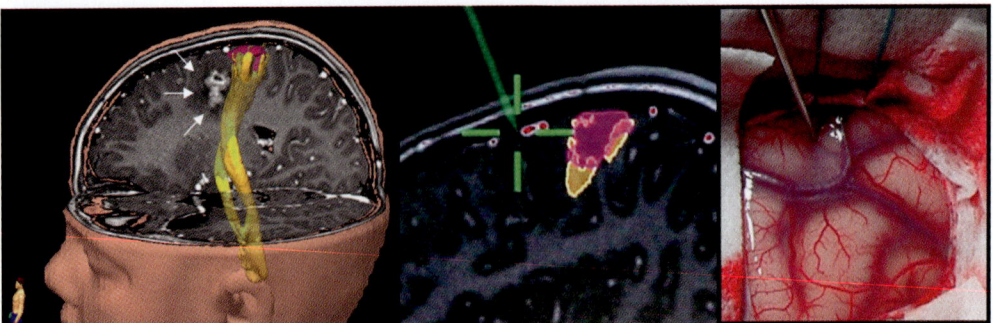

*Fig. 2. Structural MRI, fMRI and fibre tracking and their intraoperative application in a 6-year-old child with a precentral tumour. Left and central: contrast-enhanced T1-weighted images overlaid with fMRI activation during active left hand movement (pink area) and fibre tracking of the corticospinal tract (yellow area) in the vicinity of the tumour with surrounding oedema (white arrows). Intraoperative application within the neuronavigation system (evaluation and navigation with iPlan 2.6, Brainlab). The pointer of the intraoperative navigation system (right) is visualized (central image) by the green line and cross, illustrating the relation to the relevant areas.*

## Transcranial magnetic stimulation as a complementary technique in the evaluation of the sensorimotor system

fMRI always needs to be part of a set of diagnostic tools. Especially to answer the question of reorganization in the motor system, fMRI often needs transcranial magnetic stimulation (TMS) as a complementary technique. Single-pulse TMS is a noninvasive method to elicit action potential via magnetic induction in the underlying neurones. For this technique a magnetic coil is placed over the presumptive primary motor area (*e.g.*, of the hand), and a magnetic pulse is applied which leads to neuronal activation and consecutive muscle activation, measured as motor evoked potential (MEP) via self-adhesive surface electrodes to record EMGs (*e.g.*, of the first dorsal interossal muscle of both hands).

Performing TMS in children also needs careful explanation so that the child is aware of what is happening and is able to be compliant in keeping the head still. Especially in children with increased activation thresholds due to antiepileptic drugs, pre-contraction of the target muscle (by pressing the thumb to the index finger) helps to elicit motor evoked potentials. Rarely children complain about light headache after several magnetic pulses, and some are a little frightened at the beginning of the examination because the magnetic pulses come along with a clicking sound. But in general TMS is well tolerated (Garvey & Mall, 2008). Theoretically a provocation of epileptic seizures is possible, but to date this has only been reported for patients with severe epilepsy. Therefore epilepsy is a relative contraindication. In the presurgical setting, however, it is an important complementary technique, as illustrated in the following two cases.

**Case three** was a 6-year-old boy with right hemispheric dysplasia. He had hemiparesis, but grasp function of the paretic hand was preserved. Because of refractory epilepsy, he underwent presurgical evaluation, and hemispherotomy was discussed. But the question arose of whether the boy would lose function of the paretic hand after hemispherotomy because, as previously shown, dysplastic cortex can bear function (Staudt *et al.*, 2004b). To answer this question, sensorimotor fMRI (active hand movement) was done. The result for active movement of the paretic hand was activation in the ipsilateral, but not the contralateral hand-knob area. TMS of the malformed hemisphere could not elicit any response, but TMS of the contralesional hemisphere did elicit motor evoked potentials with the same short latency both in the contralateral and in the ipsilateral hand (Fig. 3) (Staudt *et al.*, 2001, 2004a, 2004b). At the age of 10 years, the boy underwent hemispherotomy, and grasp function of the paretic hand was preserved.

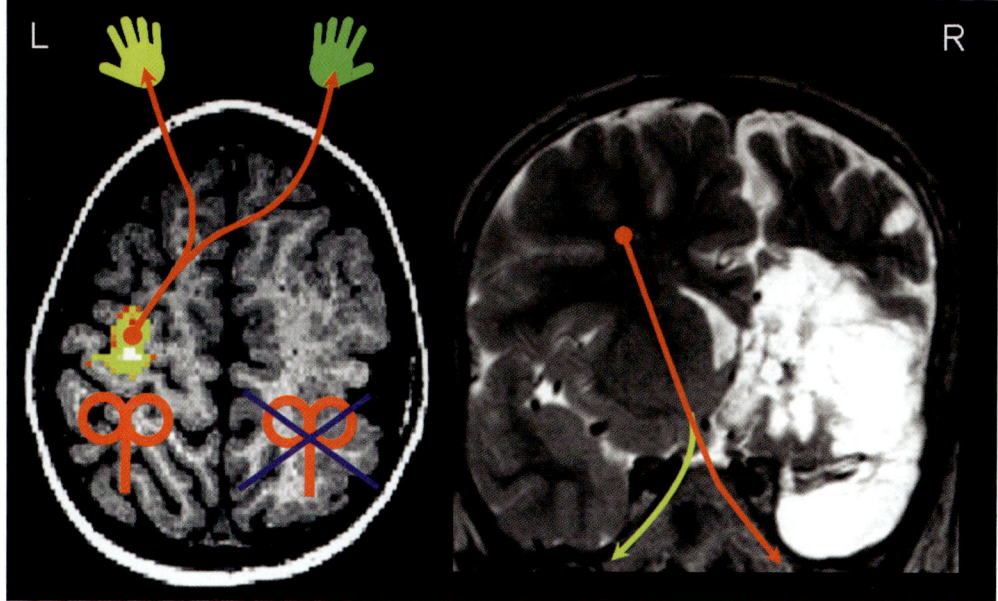

Fig. 3. TMS, fMRI of a 6-year-old child with right hemispheric dysplasia. Left: results of fMRI (yellow area = ipsilateral motor activation after active movement of the paretic hand) and TMS stimulation (pictured as an eight-shaped coil) are shown, superimposed on an axial T1 image. TMS of the contralesional hemisphere elicits contralateral (green hand, normal pattern) and ipsilateral (yellow hand, reorganization pattern) MEP. TMS of the malformed hemisphere has no effect (blue crossing). Hemispherotomy was performed without loss of grasp function. Right: postoperative T2 coronal plane together with illustration of preserved corticospinal projections.

**Case four** was an 8-year-old girl with refractory epilepsy on account of a congenital corticosubcortical infarction of the middle cerebral artery and hemiparesis with preserved grasp function of the paretic hand. Functional MRI with active movement of the paretic hand showed bilateral activation of the central (rolandic) region, which needed further evaluation. TMS of the lesioned hemisphere could not elicit any motor evoked potential, but TMS of the contralesional hemisphere showed MEPs with similar short latency in both hands. This identified the ipsilateral activation as the primary motor area (M1). The contralateral activation remained unclear. fMRI with passive movement of the paretic hand showed an exclusive contralateral activation, which was suggestive of primary somatosensory area (S1) (Fig. 4). Altogether a dissociation of the primary motor (M1) and primary somatosensory (S1) area could be shown in this patient, with ipsilateral re-organization of M1 and a normal contralateral organization of S1 (Staudt *et al.*, 2006).

### Language system

Indications for evaluating the language system are similar to those for the motor system but concern lateralization more than localization of language areas in patients with tumours or epileptogenic brain tissue and the question of re-organization.

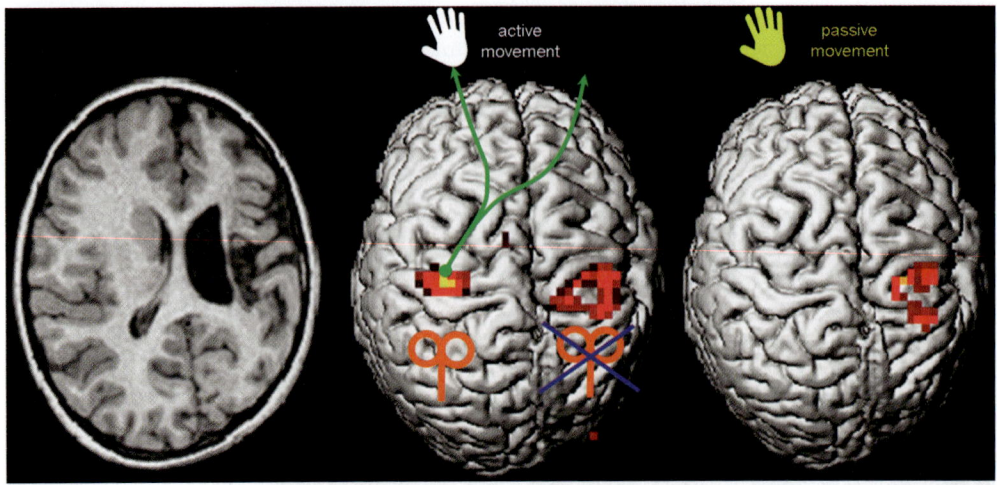

*Fig. 4. Case 4. Left: lesion after congenital infarction on axial T1 image. Middle: bilateral central fMRI activation during active movement of the paretic hand together with bilateral (green arrow-lines) MEPs (TMS symbolized with the eight-shaped coil) of the contralesional hemisphere and missing MEPs from the damaged hemisphere. Right: exclusive contralateral fMRI activation during passive movement of the paretic hand. fMRI activation superimposed on the 3D-surface brain of the patient. (Reprinted with permission from Loddenkemper & Staudt, 2010).*

Many tasks to assess perceptive and productive language function in children have been developed (*e.g.*, Gaillard *et al.*, 2004; Wilke *et al.*, 2006). Which task to use depends both on indication and on the child's capacities. In our setting the easiest task is the *beep story task*. In the 'active' condition, children just need to listen to a story in which important words are replaced by a sinus tone (beep) and, in the control condition, to a series of sinus tones. The replacement of the words by beeps was shown to activate frontal language areas in the dominant hemisphere in addition to the bilateral temporal activation (Wilke *et al.*, 2005). Another task we use is the *word generation task*, which can be performed with modifications, depending on the skills and interests of the children. In older children, the patient is given one initial word and is instructed to silently generate 'word chains' (the next word always has to begin with the final letter of the previous one), whereas smaller children create verbs to acoustical or visually presented nouns or nouns that belong to one word group (all fruits, animals, flowers, *etc.*, that the child knows). The problem with these tasks is the lack of task performance control. To overcome this, other visually presented tasks have been implemented. If children know how to read they can perform a task in which they have to decide whether two words are synonyms (*e.g.*, does rubbish = waste?) and during the control condition they have to decide whether senseless letter strings are similar (*e.g.*, MFYXRW = MFYXRW?). For children of about 5 to 6 years of age who do not yet know how to read, it is possible to present pictures together with one vowel (*e.g.*, the phoneme 'I') and let the children decide whether the presented word contains this sound (Wilke *et al.*, 2006).

Comparing results of the Wada procedure (= intracarotid amobarbital test, IAT) with fMRI results, a great concordance between both was shown (Benke *et al.*, 2006; Woermann *et al.*, 2003), especially regarding frontal fMRI activation (Deblaere *et al.*, 2004). The above-described productive language tasks elicit frontal activation; the beep story task, as a mixture of perceptive and productive language, often shows lateralized bitemporal activation together with lateralized frontal activation. In clinical practice it is helpful to have the possibility of using different productive tasks to increase the rate of successful examinations in children.

**Case five** is a-20-year-old mentally retarded woman with left hemispheric Sturge-Weber syndrome and refractory focal epilepsy. Language was one of her best skills, but because of the mental retardation and anxious personality, she was not able to undergo the stressful Wada procedure. With intensive instructions and her mother's support, however, she could undergo fMRI. The beep story task and the word chain task were done twice each (Fig. 5). In the more complex word chain task, there was no reproduced activation, but in the beep story task a reproduced right temporal activation was seen. This strongly right-lateralized activation supported the process of decision-making regarding epilepsy surgery. An anterior and posterior disconnection of the affected hemisphere was performed (in order to preserve motor function) without any effects on language.

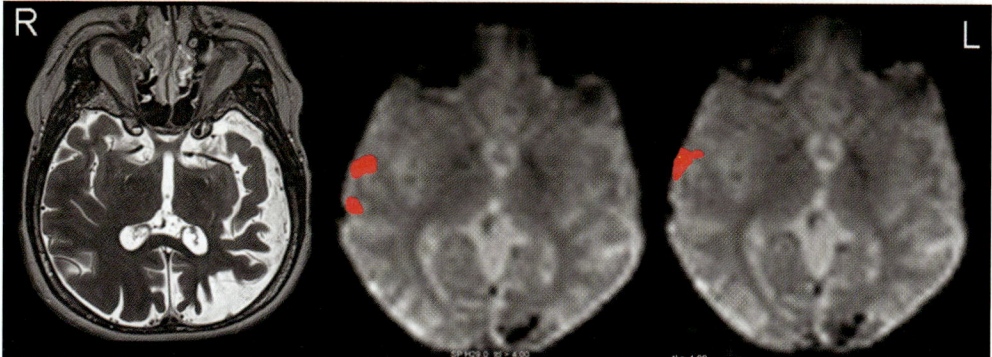

Fig. 5. Structural and functional MRI of a patient with Sturge-Weber syndrome. Left: axial T2-weighted image: atrophy of the affected hemisphere. Middle and right: reproduced lateralized right temporal activation during 'beep story task' (activation overlaid on EPI-image, threshold: T = 4).

**Case six** was a 10-year-old girl who had partial resection of a left frontal cortical dysplasia (FCD) and ongoing epilepsy. To answer the question of language lateralization, language fMRI was performed. She did several productive tasks (*e.g.*, verb generation and word generation) and the beep story task. In both (productive and perceptive tasks), the result was left lateralization of language (Fig. 6). This helped planning further procedures.

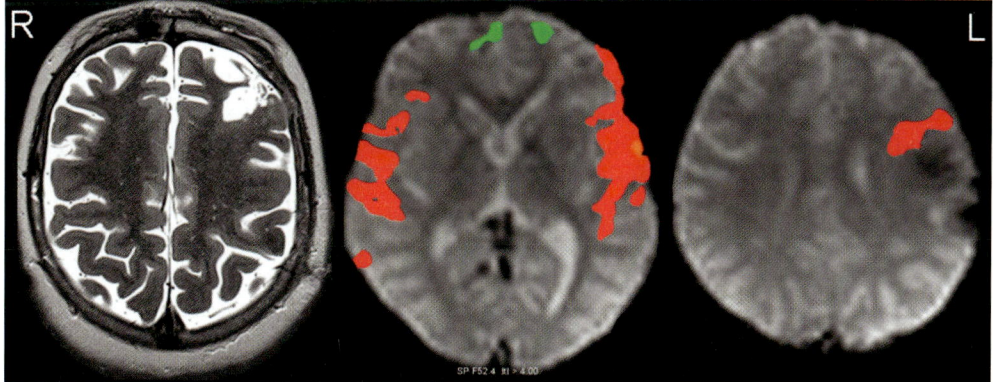

Fig. 6. Anatomic and functional images of case 6, displaying the area of previous incomplete resection of the FCD and the left-lateralized activation (red areas = activation; green areas = deactivation) both in the beep story task (middle) and the productive language tasks (right). (For both tasks threshold T = 4.)

## Visual system

FMRI can also be used to explore the visual system. In cooperative children a selective mapping of the four quadrants of the visual field is possible. Children are instructed to fixate the centre of the visual field and watch a film that is presented there. This film attracts the child's interest, helps to maintain fixation, and prevents eye movements. As shown in Fig. 7 the film is placed in the centre of a dartboard that is divided into four quadrants. While the film is shown, there is a alternating flickering of the quadrants with 4 Hz in a block design, and each quadrant is 'active' four times (Pflugfelder, 2007). In this way, it is possible to explore the activation of each quadrant separately in one examination. In noncooperative children, first reports of stimulating the visual system under sedation or anaesthesia with a bright flickering stimulus have been published (Marcar et al., 2006).

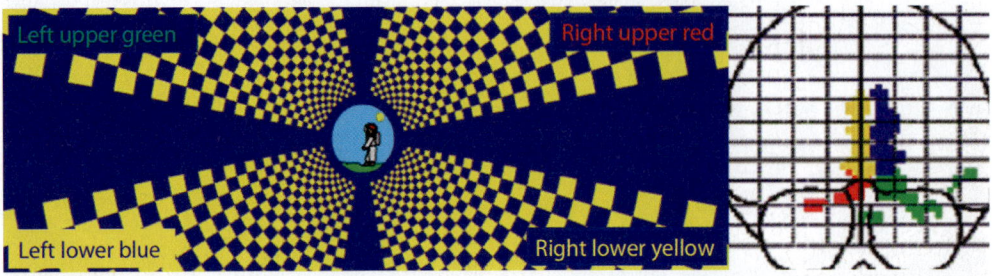

*Fig.7. Left: the visual stimulation task with the film in the centre of the dartboard. Right: visual stimulation results of healthy subjects in the frontal maximum intension projection – the four colours of the activation areas are corresponding to the stimulation as described on left image. (Modified with permission from Pflugfelder, 2007).*

**Case seven** gives an example of the retinotopic stimulation in a 16-year-old patient with a left parieto-occipital focal cortical dysplasia and refractory epilepsy. The evaluation of language and visual fMRI together with the diffusion tensor imaging of the optic radiation is shown in Fig. 8. With fMRI it was shown that there was no reorganization of the primary visual cortex and that there was no anopia due to the dysplasia.

## Conclusions

In this chapter we have demonstrated the methodology and given examples of clinical fMRI in children. The procedure was feasible even in younger children if the task was adapted to the children's skills. fMRI allows a noninvasive mapping of sensorimotor, language, and visual functions and, combined with other techniques like TMS or DTI, plays an important role in the presurgical evaluation of children.

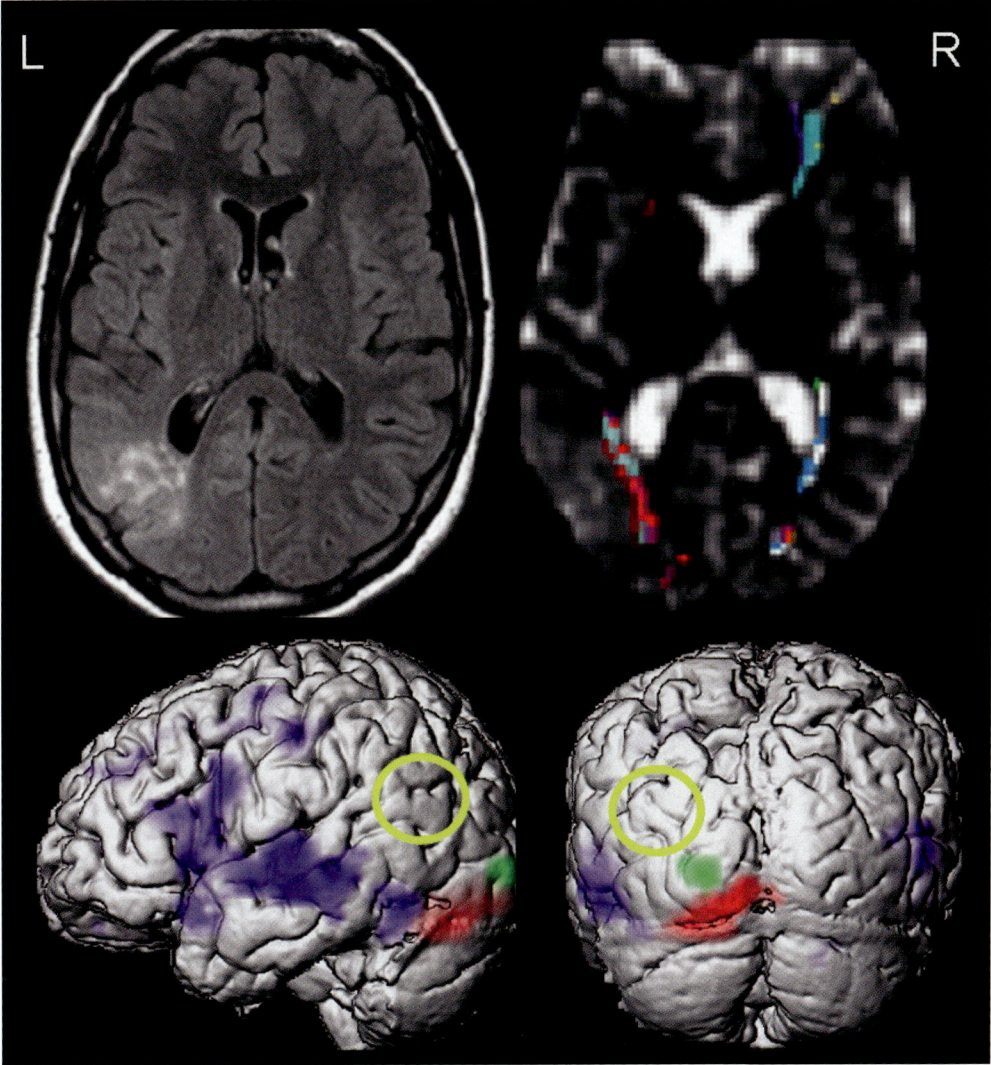

Fig. 8. Structural, DTI, and fMRI of a patient with a left parieto-occipital focal cortical dysplasia. Upper left: T2-weighted image, parieto-occipital hyperintensity reflecting the FCD in the vicinity of the optic radiation (upper right, DTI). Bottom: activation of the beep story task (blue areas) and the visual stimulation (right upper quadrant red and right lower quadrant green) on the 3D-surface brain of the patient – the area of the dysplasia is marked with the yellow circle.

## References

Benke, T., Köylü, B., Visani, P., Karner, E., Brenneis, C., Bartha, L., et al. (2006): Language lateralization in temporal lobe epilepsy: a comparison between fMRI and the Wada test. Epilepsia **47**, 1308–1319.

Carter, C.S., Heckers, S., Nichols, T., Pine, D.S. & Strother, S. (2008): Optimizing the design and analysis of clinical functional magnetic resonance imaging research studies. Biol. Psychiatr. **64**, 842–849.

Deblaere, K., Boon, P.A., Vandermaele, P. Tieleman, A., Vonck, K., Vingerhoets, G., et al. (2004): MRI language dominance assessment in epilepsy patients at 1.0 T: region of interest analysis and comparison with intracarotid amytal testing. Neuroradiology **46**, 413–420.

Gaillard, W.D., Balsalmo, L., Xu, B., McKinney, C., Papero, P.H., Weinstein, S., et al. (2004): fMRI language task panel improves determination of language dominance. *Neurology* **63**, 1403–1408.

Garvey, M.A. & Mall, V. (2008): Transcranial magnetic stimulation in children. *Clin. Neurophysiol.* **119**, 973–984.

Guzzetta, A., Staudt, M., Petacchi, E., Ehlers, J., Erb, M., Wilke, M., et al. (2007): Brain representation of active and passive hand movements in children. *Pediatric Res.* **61**, 485–490.

Loddenkemper, T. & Staudt, M. (2010): Eloquent cortex and the role of plasticity. In: *Treatment of Epilepsy* (5th ed.), eds. E. Wyllie, G.D. Cascino, B.E. Gidal & H.P. Goodkin. Philadelphia, Pennsylvania: Lippincott Williams & Wilkins.

Lotze, M., Erb, M., Flor, H., Huelsman, E., Godde, B. & Grodd, W. (2000): fMRI evaluation of somatotopic representation in human primary motor cortex. *NeuroImage* **11**, 473–481.

Marcar, V.L., Schwarz, U., Martin, E. & Lonneker, T. (2006): How depth of anesthesia influences the blood oxygenation level-dependent signal form the visual cortex of children. *Am. J. Neuroradiol.* **27**, 799–805.

Norris, D.G. (2006): Principles of magnetic resonance assessment of brain function. *J. Magn. Res. Imaging* **23**, 794–807.

Ogawa, S., Lee, T.M., Kay, A.R. & Tank, D.W. (1990): Brain magnetic resonance imaging with contrast dependent on blood oxygenation (cerebral blood flow/brain metabolism/oxygenation). *Proc. Natl. Acad. Sci. USA* **87**, 9868–9872.

Pflugfelder, A. (2007): Etablierung und Anwendung funktioneller Magnetresonanztomographie des visuellen Kortex bei Kindern. Inaugural-Dissertation Eberhards Karl Universität, Tübingen, Germany.

Staudt, M. (2010): Multimodal brain mapping in children with early brain lesions. In: *fMRI: basics and clinical applications*, eds. S. Ulmer & O. Jansen, pp 149–154. Berlin-Heidelberg: Springer Verlag.

Staudt, M., Pieper, T., Grodd, W., Winkler, P., Holthausen, H. & Krägeloh-Mann, I. (2001): Functional MRI in a 6-year-old boy with unilateral cortical malformation: concordant representation of both hands in the unaffected hemisphere. *Neuropediatrics* **32**, 159–161.

Staudt, M., Gerloff, G., Grodd, W., Holthausen, H., Niemann, G. & Krägeloh-Mann, I. (2004a): Reorganization in congenital hemiparesis acquired at different gestational ages. *Ann. Neurol.* **56**, 854–863.

Staudt, M., Krägeloh-Mann, I., Holthausen, H., Gerloff, C. & Grodd, W. (2004b): Searching for motor functions in dysgenic cortex: a clinical TMS and fMRI study. *J. Neurosurg.* **101**, 69–77.

Staudt, M., Erb, M., Holthausen, H., Grodd, W. & Krägeloh -Mann, I. (2005): Presurgical motor fMRI in a 3-year-old child [abstract]. *Neuropediatrics* **36**, 155.

Staudt, M., Braun, C., Gerloff, C., Erb, M., Grodd, W. & Krägeloh-Mann, I. (2006): Developing somatosensory projections bypass periventricular brain lesions. *Neurology* **67**, 522–525.

Wilke, M., Holland, S.K., Myseros, J.S., Schmithorst, V.J. & Ball, W.S., Jr. (2003): Functional magnetic resonance imaging in pediatrics. *Neuropediatrics* **34**, 225–233.

Wilke, M., Lidzba, K., Staudt, M., Buchenau, K., Grodd, W. & Krägeloh-Mann, I. (2005): Comprehensive language mapping in children, using functional magnetic resonance imaging: what's missing counts. *NeuroReport* **16**, 915–919.

Wilke, M., Lidzba, K., Staudt, M., Buchenau, K., Grodd, W. & Krägeloh-Mann, I. (2006): An fMRI task battery for assessing hemispheric language dominance in children. *NeuroImage* **32**, 400–410.

Woermann, F.G., Jokir, H., Luerding, M.S., Freitag, H., Schulz, R., Guertler, S., et al. (2003): Language lateralization by Wada test and fMRI in 100 patients with epilepsy. *Neurology* **61**, 699–701.

## Chapter 11

# Clinical and instrumental assessment of the upper limb in cerebral palsy

Giuseppina Sgandurra[*,§] and Giovanni Cioni[§,o]

[*]Scuola Superiore Sant'Anna, piazza Martiri della Libertà 33, 56127 Pisa, Italy;
[§]Department of Developmental Neuroscience, Stella Maris Scientific Institute, via dei Giacinti 2, 56128 Calambrone, Pisa, Italy;
[o]Division of Child Neurology and Psychiatry, University of Pisa, Pisa, Italy
gsgandurra@inpe.unipi.it
gcioni@inpe.unipi.it

### Summary

Upper limbs are effective tools that are used in many necessary tasks of daily life, and their function is complex and influenced by many factors. Children with cerebral palsy (CP) are faced with a variety of motor and sensory impairments that have an impact on the functioning of their arms. Several clinical and instrumental tools are available to assess the upper limbs in CP, and it is important that the clinician be prepared to examine and choose tools carefully for the task at hand, with due regard to the psychometric properties of each measure, such as validity, reliability, and responsiveness. Furthermore, in recent years, new instrumental assessments of the upper limb have been developed that are useful in understanding the developmental process in healthy children and in differentiating distinct levels of impairment in children with neurologic disorders. In this review we have discussed some classifications of hand function (Manual Ability Classification System, House's and Ferrari's classification), revised the psychometric properties of many clinical scales (Ashworth), Quality of Upper Extremity Skills Test, Jebsen–Taylor Hand Function Test, Melbourne Assessment, Assisting Hand Assessment, Goal Attainment Scale, ABILHAND-Kids, Paediatric Evaluation of Disability Inventory, and Canadian Occupational Performance Measure) and have mentioned some instrumental assessments (kinematic and electrophysiologic analyses). The methods used to assess hand function are multifaceted, and a single universal instrument does not exist. Combining information from valid clinical and instrumental measurements can improve the understanding of hand function, treatment planning, and measurement of real changes.

### Introduction

The upper limbs are effective tools that are used in the multiple tasks of daily life. Their function is complex and influenced by many factors. The successful performance of manual skills depends on a complex of processes that include the cognitive, somatosensory, perceptual, and musculoskeletal systems. Cognition and related components (motivation, attention, and concentration) are very important because one has to understand the value of using one's hand for a meaningful purpose and to be motivated to perform it. The integration of somatosensory information is crucial for the fine tuning of motor commands, force regulation, and the build-up of memory strategies for grasping and manipulating the objects. The perceptual system provides information about the position of the hand in space, as well as the position of the target. Finally, musculoskeletal components are crucial for motor output (Eliasson, 2005). Cerebral palsy (CP) describes 'a group of disorders of the development of movement and posture, causing activity limitation' that are attributed to non-progressive disturbance that occurred in the developing foetal or infant brain. The motor disorders of CP are often accompanied by disturbance of sensation, cognition, communication, perception, and/or behaviour, and or by seizure disorder (Bax *et al.*, 2005). Therefore, children with CP are faced with a variety of motor and sensory impairments that have an impact on their arm's functioning (Uvebrant, 1988), and these problems can be approached and understood from a variety of angles. Krumlinde-Sundholm (2008) states that 'the methods used to assess hand function are multifaceted and it would be terrific to have one universal tool, something corresponding to a Swiss army knife, which could be used for needs and which simply assess hand function. Unfortunately, a single universal instrument does not exist. Instead we need to carefully select the right tool for the task we wish to evaluate and address in intervention.' It is therefore essential that we be clear about what we wish to accomplish before beginning to measure and then to find the tools that will enable us to reach that goal. It is important to ascertain that a measure is valid for the purpose for which it is being used, so it should be clear that the measure is actually capable of determining that specific goal. Even well-developed and validated measures may not be able to aid in tasks for which they were not specifically created and validated. Consequently, the user of clinical assessment measures must be prepared to examine and choose tools carefully for the task at hand with due regard to the properties of each measure (Rosenbaum, 1998).

## Clinical tests

**Measurement properties**

There are two main types of standardized tests: *norm-referenced* and *criterion-referenced*. In the norm-referenced tests, the child's performance is compared to the average performance of typically developed age-matched peers, which constitutes a normative sample. The most important contribution of these tests for children with disabilities is their use in identifying the child's needs and eligibility for therapy services by determining the extent of the child's delay or dysfunction. However, their results will not be useful for detecting changes over time (Hanna, *et al.*, 2005). Instead, criterion-referenced scores are interpreted by considering directly whether children can do specific tasks that are important for their age, grade, or clinical context. By means of these tests, improvement in skills may be captured and the child's change over time will be measured in relation to himself (Krumlinde-Sundholm, 2008). In addition, there are three main purposes for which standardized tests in general are constructed (Boyce *et al.*, 1991; Rosenbaum, 1998), depending on whether the measure is to be used for discriminating among subjects (discriminative or descriptive measures), predicting subject outcomes (screening or predictive measures), or evaluating change over time (evaluative measures). Although it is possible for a measure to satisfy more than one purpose, each of these functions should be validated separately. To be useful, a test needs to fulfil some basic criteria concerning psychometric properties, such as validity, reliability, and responsiveness. Furthermore, information about standard error measure (SEM) or the smallest detectable difference (SDD) is important for interpreting the change in individuals. Hanna *et al.* (2005) have created the 'Clinical

Measurement Practical Guidelines for Service Providers', available on the website for the CanChild Centre for Childhood Disability Research to clearly explain the measures' psychometric properties and how to interpret them (www.canchild.ca/en/canchildresources/resources/ClinicalMeasurement.pdf).

**International Classification of Functioning, Disability and Health framework**

In addition to the purpose of a measure (*why* we measure), it is also important to know *what* we measure, which is possible using an organizing framework. The International Classification of Functioning, Disability and Health (ICF) is a classification system developed by the World Health Organization (WHO, 2001) that provides a framework for measuring and documenting health outcomes. The 2001 version for adults was followed in 2007 by an ICF for children and youth (WHO, 2007). The components of ICF are (i) body functions (*i.e.*, physiologic and psychological functions of the body system) and body structures (*i.e.*, the anatomic construct of the body); (ii) activities (*e.g.*, the execution of tasks or actions by individuals); (iii) participation (*e.g.*, involvement in life situations); (iv) environmental factors (*e.g.*, the physical, social, and attitudinal situations in which people live); (v) personal factors (*e.g.*, the particular background of individuals' life and living situation).

Within this model, the human (and individual) experience of functioning is not considered as the consequence of a disease, but the result of the interaction between a health condition and both personal attributes and environmental influences. Another factor that emerges from the ICF is the differentiation between the qualifiers of capacity and performance. Capacity refers to the child's ability to execute a task (for hand function, *e.g.*, to grasp, transport, or press) on the highest probable level of functioning that the child may reach in a standardized environment. The performance qualifier describes what an individual actually does in his or her current environment (*e.g.*, spontaneous use of the upper limbs during activities or play), and so brings in the aspect of a person's involvement in life situations. Clinical measures, therefore, need to be multidimensional in order to encompass functioning at different levels of the ICF (Rosenbaum & Stewart, 2004). No single tool covers all domains of the ICF, and many authors have started to carefully analyze and code each item in the assessment according to it (Cieza *et al.*, 2005; Gilmore *et al.*, 2009; Krumlinde-Sundholm, 2008). Many outcome measures in current use are fairly specific for one domain of the ICF, while others may span two or more domains. Actually, a range of tools is required to comprehensively assess hand function in children with CP. Choosing the most appropriate outcome measures or assessment tools in clinical research for the clinical care of CP is challenging (Vargus-Adams, 2009). To help clinicians in the field of paediatric rehabilitation to select the most appropriate outcome measures with demonstrated reliability, validity, clinical responsiveness, and clinical utility a software called All About Outcomes© has been developed by investigators at CanChild (Law *et al.*, 1999).

**Classifications of hand function**

Classifications are useful to describe and to group people who have similar characteristics. Because classifications do not include detailed descriptions, they are not intended to measure or detect change, especially when the behaviours classified are complex. The purpose of a classification system is simply to describe common characteristics and to increase communication between professionals (Krumlinde-Sundholm, 2008). However, some classifications, such as that of House, were used to detect changes.

## Manual Ability Classification System

The Manual Ability Classification System (MACS) (www.MACS.nu) aims to describe the manual ability of children with CP when they are handling objects in daily activities. It is constructed on five levels: level I indicates the best and level V the lowest level of manual ability. The level is determined by asking someone who knows the child about his or her typical performance and need for help in handling objects. It can be used in children from 4 to 18 years of age and has shown good reliability and validity. It has demonstrated an excellent inter-observer reliability between health professionals, with an intra-class correlation coefficient (ICC) of 0.97. There is a perfect agreement between families and professionals for more than 50 per cent of children; the indices of chance-corrected agreement ranged from $\kappa = 0.3$ to 0.5, and the reliability coefficients ranged from ICC 0.7 to 0.9 (Eliasson *et al.*, 2006b; Morris *et al.*, 2006; Rosenbaum & Stewart; 2004). It has already been translated into 14 languages, including Italian.

## House classification system

The House classification (House *et al.*, 1981) has been developed for the evaluation of function in the affected hand after surgery for thumb-in-palm deformity in children with spastic hemiplegic CP and has been used to evaluate children before and after upper extremity botulinum toxin injections (Hoare *et al.*, 2010). Even if it is constructed for hemiplegic CP, in some studies it is used for each hand separately in all types of CP by observing the child in activities requiring bimanual hand function (Arner *et al.*, 2008). The classification consists of nine grades ranging from a hand that is not used at all (grade 0) to one that is used spontaneously and independently of the other hand (grade 8). Commonly, to obtain good agreement, the classification is divided in four groups: no use (0), passive assist (1–3), active assist (4–6), or spontaneous use (7–8). With these four groups it is shown that inter-observer reliability is good ($\kappa$ value 0.54) and intra-observer reliability is excellent ($\kappa$ value 0.80) (Waters *et al.*, 2004). Recently, Koman *et al.* (2008) have proposed a new version of the House classification called the Modified House Functional Classification (MHC) system. In this study, the addition of 32 yes/no modifiers to the original system resulted in an instrument with excellent inter- and intra-rater reliability. MHC involves the observation of patients during the performance of increasingly complex functional activities. Inter-rater agreement (ICC = 0.94) and intra-rater agreement (ICC = 0.96) on the MHC is good to excellent.

## Classification of manipulation by Ferrari and collaborators

In recent years our group has attempted to validate a classification of hand function applicable to children with spastic hemiplegic CP (Cioni *et al.*, 2009; Ferrari & Cioni, 2005). It describes five patterns of manipulation (integrated, semi-functional, synergic, imprisoned, and excluded hand) by analyzing hand kinematic profile and functional use. The manipulation skills of 35 children and adolescents (age range, 4–15 years) with hemiplegic CP were studied among patients whose videos were stored in the archives of the Department of Developmental Neuroscience of the IRCCS Stella Maris (Pisa, Italy) and of the Children's Rehabilitation Unit of S. Maria Nuova Hospital (Reggio Emilia, Italy). The results were blindly scored at first by two of the authors of the classification (defined as 'maximum experts'), then by 10 expert observers who performed test-retest (after 4 months). Finally, the 35 videos in which the highest agreement was reached by 10 scores were later classified by 124 rehabilitation professionals after a training course on the classification. High kappa [$\kappa$] values (range, 0.836–0.982) were obtained for test-retest of the 10 expert observers, whereas a substantial agreement ($\kappa = 0.70$) was found in the group of 124 scorers. In the same sample of 35 cases, the external validity was also determined by correlating hand manipulation classes with scores of the Melbourne Assessment of Unilateral Upper Limb Function. The regression coefficient was very high (R = 0.86), indicating a significant correlation between the two scales. Also, our group (Perazza *et al.*, 2008) has tested the external validity correlating hand manipulation classes with the House classification. A high concordance for classification of manipulation (ICC, 0.996; Fleiss' kappa, 0.93; Spearman rho coefficient intraoperator, 0.986; Spearman rho coefficient between two operators and gold standard, 0.996 and 0.989, respectively, $p < 0.01$) and for the House scale (ICC,0.994; Fleiss' kappa, 0.86; Spearman rho coefficient intraoperator, 0.981; Spearman rho coefficient between two operators and gold standard, 0.982 and 0.986, respectively, $p < 0.01$) was found. Lastly, R square between the two scales was 0.887, indicating a high linear correlation.

### Ashworth scale and Modified Ashworth Scale

The scale proposed by Ashworth (1964) is a five-point rating criterion-referenced ordinal scale for measuring muscle tone with ratings from 0 ('no increase in tone') to 4 ('limb rigid in flexion or extension'). Because Bohannon and Smith (1987), in an early investigation of its reliability, found a clustering of scores at its lower end, they added an extra item to the lower end (grade 1+). This new version is called the Modified Ashworth Scale (MAS). According to the ICF, the Ashworth scale and MAS measure the impairment of body function (Fig.1). The intra-rater reliability of MAS is from 0.55 to 0.83 and the inter-rater reliability from 0.45 to 0.84 (Morris, 2002). These estimations have been supported in recent studies in children with CP where inter-rater reliability has been described as low (Fosang, *et al.*, 2003; Yam & Leung, 2006). The MAS has demonstrated changes in children after injection of botulinum toxin A (BTX-A) into the upper limb combined with occupational therapy (Hoare *et al.*, 2010).

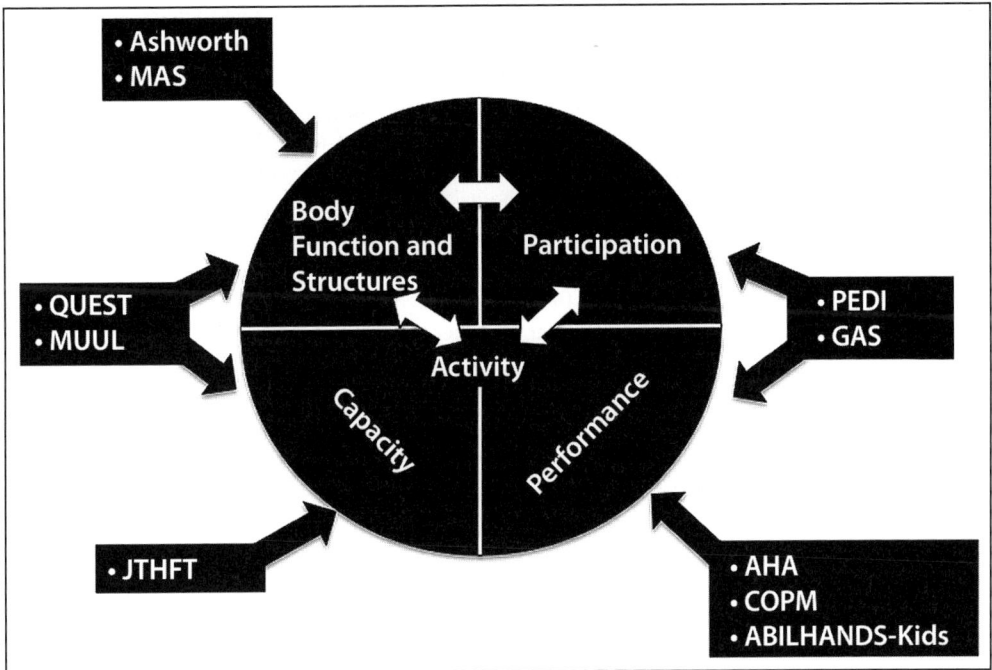

*Fig. 1. Clinical tests for hand function in children, classified according to the International Classification of Functioning, Disability and Health (ICF). MAS: Modified Ashworth Scale; QUEST: Quality of Upper Extremity Skills Test; JTHFT: Jebsen-Taylor Hand Function Test; MUUL: Melbourne Assessment of Unilateral Upper Limb Function; AHA: Assisting Hand Assessment; GAS: Goal Attainment Scale; PEDI: Paediatric Evaluation of Disability Inventory; COPM: Canadian Occupational Performance Measure.*

## Quality of Upper Extremity Skills Test

The Quality of Upper Extremity Skills Test (QUEST) is a descriptive, impairment-based and evaluative measure designed to evaluate movement patterns and hand function in children with CP separately for each arm (DeMatteo et al., 1993). The purpose of the QUEST is to evaluate within a play context the quality of upper extremity function in 36 items subvided into four domains: dissociated movement, grasp, protective extension, and weight bearing. Each item is scored with a dichotomous scale as either a pass or a fail or else not-tested. According to the ICF, the QUEST measures the child's capacity in the domain of activity with the grasps subscale, and the impairment of body function with the dissociated movement subscales (Fig.1) (Klingels et al., 2010). Validation studies have been completed with children with CP, aged 18 months to 8 years. Variable intra-rater reliability (ranges from 0.51 to 0.96 with all coefficients except one greater than 0.70) and strong test-retest reliability (ranges from 0.75 to 0.95) have been reported (Haga et al., 2007; Sorsdahl et al., 2008). Gilmore et al. (2009) suggested that this discrepancy may be a result of small numbers of raters and depends on which round of assessment scores was used to determine the inter-rater reliability. The QUEST has frequently been used in clinical trials that investigate the effects of BTX-A injections and it was responsive to changes in quality of movement after upper extremity casting (Hoare et al., 2010). The SDD is 7.1 per cent. The QUEST can be administered and scored within 45 minutes.

## Jebsen–Taylor Hand Function Test

The Jebsen–Taylor Hand Function Test (JTHFT) is a short unimanual test to score movement speed during seven unimanual tasks. It was developed by Jebsen et al. (1969) to evaluate adults with neurologic or musculoskeletal conditions involving hand disabilities. The test includes seven items, which are timed: (1) writing (copying) a 24-letter sentence; (2) turning over cards; (3) picking up small common objects such as a paper clip, bottle cap, and coin; (4) simulated feeding using a teaspoon and five kidney beans; (5) stacking checkers; (6) picking up large light objects; and (7) picking up large heavy objects. The test takes approximately 15 minutes to complete, but can take up to 45 minutes with slower patients. In studies of children with CP the handwriting task was omitted and the maximum allowable time of each task was reduced to 2 minutes to limit frustration (Charles et al., 2006; Sakzewski et al., 2010). Normative data are available for males and females in the 20–60 year age range, for both the dominant and nondominant hand (Jebsen et al., 1969). The test has been used with children 6 years or older and is also a measure of speed and dexterity (Eliasson et al., 2006a; Taylor et al., 1973); however, psychometric data reported for children with hemiplegia are not available (Sakzewski et al., 2010). According to the ICF, the JTHFT measures the capacity in the domain of activity (Fig.1) (Klingels et al., 2010).

## Melbourne Assessment of Unilateral Upper Limb Function

The Melbourne Assessment of Unilateral Upper Limb Function (MUUL) is an evaluative tool that measures unilateral upper extremity quality of movement in children aged from 5 to 15 years with neurologic impairments (Randall et al., 1999, 2001). A modified MUUL for children 2 to 4 years of age has recently been developed (Randall et al., 2008). MUUL is a criterion-referenced test based on 16 items scored on a 3- to 5-point ordinal scale and comprising tasks that are representative of the most important components of unilateral upper limb function (reaching, grasping, releasing, and manipulation). Most items are further subdivided into two to four sub-items (for a total of 37 sub-items) that represent an aspect of the required movement, such as range of movement, fluency, target accuracy, speed, and quality of movement. The total score can range from 0 to 122 points and can be converted to a percentage. According to the ICF, the MUUL measures both capacity in the domain of activity and some aspects at the body functional level (*e.g..* range of motion, fluency) (Fig. 1) (Klingels *et al.*, 2010). The test is administered with the child's performance recorded on videotape for subsequent scoring. The inter-rater reliability (ICC) for the total score is 0.97. Percentage of agreement of the sub-items varied between 35 and 95 per cent. The intra-rater reliability was also high (ICC 0.97) (Klingels *et al.*, 2008). In the first reliability study of MUUL, Randall *et al.* (2001) demonstrated that when two assessments of the same child, scored by the same therapist, differ by more than 14.3 points (12 per cent), that probably reflects a true change in function rather than an error in measurement. Recently, Klingels *et al.* (2008) demonstrated that the SDD is 8.99 per cent instead of 12 per cent. The MUUL has been used in several intervention studies (Speth *et al.*, 2005; Wallen *et al.*, 2004, 2007), but some of these studies have suggested that the MUUL might not be sufficiently sensitive to changes brought about by BTX-A treatment, because the SDD was smaller than recommended and thus further investigation is warranted (Hoare *et al.*, 2010).

**Assisting Hand Assessment**

The Assisting Hand Assessment (AHA, version 4.4) is a standardized, criterion-referenced and performance-based test for use with children aged 18 months to 12 years, who have a unilateral upper limb impairment (Krumlinde-Sundholm & Eliasson, 2003; Krumlinde-Sundholm *et al.*, 2007). It evaluates the spontaneous use of the assisting hand during a semistructured play session with specific toys (from the AHA test kit) requiring bimanual handling (Fig. 1). The play context is age-appropriate, that is, there is one context for children 18 months to 5 years old (Small Kids AHA) and others (two different board games) for children aged 6–12 years (School Kids AHA). The forms are directly comparable, as demonstrated by a test-retest of alternate forms of AHA (Holmefur *et al.*, 2007). There is a new research version for children over 12 years of age (Holmstrom *et al.*, 2010). The AHA is video-taped in a standardized manner, and the play session lasts 10–15 minutes. The 22 items defining different actions are then scored on a 4-point scale rating the quality of the performance. The subsequent scoring procedures have a raw sum score range from 22 (low ability) to 88 (high ability) and a logit measure from −10.18 to +8.70. The AHA can only be administered and scored by a certified rater. Inter-rater, intra-rater, and test-retest reliability of the AHA have high ICC (0.99 and 0.98, for the small-kids and for the school-kids version, respectively) (Holmefur *et al.*, 2007; Klingels *et al.*, 2010). The smallest detectable difference (SDD) over time indicates that a change in AHA scores from one test session to the next must be 3.65 sum scores (0.76 logits) for the school kids and 3.89 sum scores (0.97 logits) for the small kids AHA (Holmefur *et al.*, 2007). The scale responsiveness to change was demonstrated in intervention studies focusing on forced-use therapy (Willis *et al.*, 2002), constraint-induced movement therapy (CIMT) (Eliasson *et al.*, 2005; Klingels *et al.*, 2010; Wallen *et al.*, 2008), hand-arm bimanual intensive therapy (HABIT) (Gordon *et al.*, 2007) and, recently, modified CIMT followed by task-specific training of goal-directed bimanual play and self-care activities (Aarts *et al.*, 2010).

**Goal Attainment Scale**

The Goal Attainment Scale (GAS) is an individualized, criterion-referenced measure of treatment-induced change. The GAS aims to measure an individual's success in achieving functional goals that have been determined prior to a treatment intervention. It is commonly used in paediatric rehabilitation to evaluate patients' and families' progress towards activity and participation goals (Fig.1). (Steenbeek et al., 2010). In its original form, it is a 5-point scale, constructed before an intervention period from −2 (current level of performance, that is, no change), −1 (less than expected outcome), 0 (expected outcome), +1 (more than expected outcome) to +2 (much greater than expected outcome). The GAS has been used in 5 of 10 RCTs evaluating the use of BTX-A and occupational therapy in children with CP, making it the most commonly used outcome measure across these trials (Hoare et al., 2010). Despite its popularity and reported sensitivity to detect change that is assumed to be better than that of standardized functional measures, the validity and reliability of the method of scale development (content reliability) and the reliability of the scores (inter-rater reliability) is largely unknown (Steenbeek et al., 2010). The reliability of GAS may be affected by the risk of so-called therapist bias such as the therapists' expectations about their patients' level of attainment for each GAS scale. With regard to sensitivity to change, Steenbeek et al. (2010) report that the responsiveness of GAS 'depends on whether therapists and parents select goals and levels of attainment for each goal that represent clinically important changes in future performance'.

## ABILHAND-Kids

The ABILHAND-Kids is a short condition-specific questionnaire that measures 21 mainly bimanual daily activities referred to the activity domain of the ICF (Fig.1) (Klingels et al., 2010). The difficulty experienced by the child to perform the required tasks is scored by a parent on a 3-point ordinal scale (impossible, difficult, easy). It has been validated and calibrated in children with CP (age 6–15) and has a high reliability ($R = .94$) and a good reproducibility over time ($R = .91$). The questionnaire was developed using the Rasch measurement model (Arnould et al., 2004). In a recent study about a modified CIMT followed by task-specific training of goal-directed bimanual play and self-care activities in children with hemiplegic CP, it demonstrated a high-effect size (Cohen's d: 1.01) (Aarts et al., 2010; Klingels et al., 2010). The ABILHAND-Kids has excellent clinical utility, being available free online, complete with online analysis of data. It is quick to administer and is completed by parents, giving a different perspective on children's manual ability in their everyday life (Gilmore et al., 2009).

## Paediatric Evaluation of Disability Inventory

The Paediatric Evaluation of Disability Inventory (PEDI) is a standardized assessment that quantifies a child's level of ability and dependency in many daily activities (Haley et al., 1992). The PEDI is designed to measure a child's abilities across three measurement scales: functional skills, caregiver assistance, and modifications used. Each scale is divided into three domains of self-care, mobility, and social function, each of which can be administered separately. For each domain, functional skills are rated dichotomously, with 0 indicating inability to perform a task and 1 indicating that a child is capable of performing the task. Caregiver assistance is rated on a 6-point ordinal scale ranging from 'total assistance' to 'independence'. It has been standardized for children aged 6 months to 7.5 years without impairment and has established reliability and validity to detect the presence, extent, and area of a functional delay in children with physical impairment or combined physical and cognitive impairment (Gilmore et al., 2009; Klingels et al., 2010). Generally for the upper limb function assessment and outcome evaluation, only self-care domain both for functional skills (73 items) and caregiver assistance (8 items) are tested. That evaluation covers a broad domain of the ICF (Fig. 1). PEDI scale construction was developed using the Rasch measurement model. High intra-rater reliability has been reported for self-care functional skills (ICCs 0.97–0.99) and self-care caregiver assistance (ICCs 0.94–0.99) (Berg et al., 2004). Iyer et al. (2003) reported that change scores of 11.5 per cent on the total scale appeared to represent clinically meaningful change. Recently, a review evaluating upper limb injection of BTX-A in children with CP, with or without occupational therapy, did not demonstrate a significant difference between groups (Hoare et al., 2010).

## Canadian Occupational Performance Measure

The Canadian Occupational Performance Measure (COPM) is a family-centred measure that lists the problems experienced in daily life through a semistructured interview. It was designed to detect change in a person's perception of his or her occupational performance in self-care abilities, productivity, and leisure activities (Fig. 1) (Law et al., 1998). Cusick et al. (2007) proposed an adapted form for very young children (aged 2–8 years) by deleting paid/unpaid work and household management categories and having parents act as proxies to rate the child's performance and their own satisfaction. Generally, five of the most important areas are selected and then scored by the parents at two levels: (i) perception of current performance (COPM-P); and (ii) satisfaction with current performance (COPM-S). The COPM ratings are on a 10-point scale; scores closer to 10 indicate better performance and increased satisfaction. It has adequate validity and adequate test-retest reliability (ICC of 0.73 for performance and 0.83 for satisfaction). The COPM has shown responsiveness to change in studies evaluating BTX-A and occupational therapy in children with CP (Hoare et al., 2010). There is evidence that a change in summary scores (*i.e.*, between initial and subsequent scores) of two or more is clinically significant (Carswell et al., 2004, Sakzewski et al., 2007).

## Instrumental assessments

Different technologies now are available for investigating hand function. They include kinematic analysis and electrophysiologic assessment such as transcranial magnetic stimulation (TMS).

## Kinematic analysis

Three-dimensional motion analysis represents a powerful instrument for a quantitative assessment in human movement analysis. It is noninvasive and provides quantitative and three-dimensional data as for kinematics (such as trajectories, velocity, accelerations, and angles), kinetics (such as forces, joint moments, and joint powers) and when associated with electromyography also offers a quantitative evaluation of muscle activity. The clinical use of gait laboratories is rapidly increasing, which aids in the diagnostic and surgical planning in lower limb treatment of children with CP. The variety, complexity, and range of upper limb movements present a big challenge to assessment and interpretation of data. The nature of free arm movements is completely different from those that are restricted, repeatable or cyclic as compared to gait. Analysis of the upper extremities is at an early stage, and its introduction to the clinical routine seems to be a step for the future (Rau et al., 2000). In our laboratory (IRCCS Stella Maris), Coluccini et al. (2007) have investigated the performance of the upper limb during the execution of functional tasks (*e.g.* reaching, grasping, and transporting and releasing of objects) in a group of healthy children and in children with motor disabilities (hemiplegic CP [HCP] and dyskinetic movement disorders [MD]). The kinematics of the upper limb were assessed using an optoelectronic motion analysis system (BTS) equipped with eight infrared cameras operating at 100 fps. The quantitative assessment was performed considering temporal duration, the amplitude of movements at different joints, and the periodicity of the acceleration patterns. Compared to adults, healthy children showed increased motion amplitudes both at the head and at the trunk; this is suggestive of a reduced ability to stabilize the head during reaching. Furthermore, healthy children showed a reduced periodicity of acceleration patterns, which is interpreted as an indication of the ongoing maturation process of the central nervous system. Subjects with HCP and MD showed increased movement duration; however, this general finding does not account for specific differences. Indeed, children with HCP showed reduced range of motion of the shoulder on the frontal plane, which is counterbalanced by the introduction of compensatory movements of the trunk. Conversely, in children with MD, the range of motion is well-preserved, whereas the movements of the head are increased, especially at higher speed. Finally, the periodicity of the end-effect is dramatically reduced, both in HCP and MD. This suggests the existence of out-of-phase corrective strokes that may indicate an increased variability of the motor control commands. Other studies about the development of precision grip have been performed by Forssberg et al. (1991, 1992) as the coupling of grip force and load force generation. Their apparatus separately measured the grip force at each surface (thumb and index finger) by strain gauge transducers, while the total load force was recorded by another strain gauge system. The vertical movement was recorded by a camera containing a light-sensitive photo-resistor sensing the position of an infrared light-emitting diode attached to the object. These authors demonstrated that young children generate grip force and load force in a sequential rather than in a parallel manner. Compared to that in adults, the duration of the preload phase was three times longer in infants younger than 10 months of age and about twice as long in children younger than 3 years old. Smaller children required several touches of the object before a stable grasp was established and also displayed longer latencies between the first and second contact. The same experiment was performed in children with CP, in whom it was shown that force rates were not produced in mainly bell-shaped curves, but rather in profiles that are step-wise, irregular, and extremely variable (Eliasson et al., 1991; Forssberg et al., 1991). The studies reported are only illustrative of the importance of kinematic and instrumental analyses of the upper limb to understand the developmental process in healthy children and to differentiate distinct levels of impairment in children with neurologic disorders.

**Transcranial magnetic stimulation**

Transcranial magnetic stimulation (TMS) is a method for focal brain stimulation based on the principle of electromagnetic induction, where small intracranial electric currents are generated by a powerful, rapidly changing extracranial magnetic field. In recent years it has provided insights into both typical neuromotor maturation and the mechanisms underlying the motor hand skill deficits in children with developmental disabilities, particularly with respect to the development of crossed and uncrossed corticospinal motor pathways (Frye et al., 2008). Eyre (2003) reported that TMS evokes bilateral arm motor effects (in both distal and proximal muscles) in both preterm and term-born infants. The amplitude of the ipsilateral effects diminished over the first year of life, and there was a parallel increase in amplitude of contralateral effects. TMS has also provided the neurophysiologic understanding of sensorimotor reorganization after early brain injuries (Eyre et al., 2007). The main mechanism for a reconnection of the motor cortex to the spinal cord consists of a reorganization within the ipsilesional cortex, based on the partial sparing of primary motor cortex or on the possibility that functions may be taken over by intact non-primary motor areas within the damaged hemisphere (ipsilesional reorganization). However, when the lesion occurs at an early stage of development, either during intrauterine life or soon after birth, a different mechanism can also be observed. It is based on the persistence of a significant component of monosynaptic fast-conducting ipsilateral motor projections; these normally withdraw within the first months of life, but may be permanently maintained if brain damage occurs early in life. In this case, the unaffected hemisphere directly controls both upper limbs, giving rise to a pattern of reorganization unknown to adult pathology (contralesional reorganization). Our group of investigators (Guzzetta et al., 2007) has recently provided some evidence indicating how, in patients with early brain damage, the pattern of sensorimotor reorganization (ipsilesional vs. contralesional) is already determined during the first year of life, and possibly even within the first few months. We also have shown that when grouping patients according to type of sensorimotor reorganization, a clear-cut segregation of the results of the MUUL was apparent, as individuals with ipsilesional reorganization scored above 80, whereas those with contralesional motor reorganization had poorly efficient motor function, only reaching a score of 70 or below. Recently, with a study using TMS and AHA, Holmstrom et al. (2010) also demonstrated that the most favourable hand function was seen in children with ipsilesional reorganization, while those with contralesional reorganization had the most impaired function. Nevertheless, in this last subgroup some children had fairly good bimanual ability, suggesting that an ipsilateral pattern can be associated with a good assisting hand (AHA 29–59 per cent).

## Conclusions

There are several clinical and instrumental tools to assess the upper limbs in cerebral palsy. In this review we have discussed many measurements, but they are only a part of those that are available. The methods used to assess hand function are multifaceted, and a single universal instrument does not exist. Combining information from valid clinical and instrumental measurements can improve the understanding of hand function, the planning of treatment, and the measurement of real changes.

## References

Aarts, P.B., Jongerius, P.H., Geerdink, Y.A., van Limbeek, J. & Geurts, A.C. (2010): Effectiveness of modified constraint-induced movement therapy in children with unilateral spastic cerebral palsy: a randomized controlled trial. *Neurorehabil. Neural Repair* **24**, 509–518.

Arner, M., Eliasson, A.C., Nicklasson, S., Sommerstein, K. & Hägglund, G. (2008): Hand function in cerebral palsy: report of 367 children in a population-based longitudinal health care program. *J. Hand Surg. Am.* **33**, 1337–1347.

Arnould, C., Penta, M., Renders, A. & Thonnard, J.L. (2004): ABILHAND-Kids: a measure of manual ability in children with cerebral palsy. *Neurology* **63**, 1045–1052.

Ashworth, B. (1964): Preliminary trial of carisoprodol in multiple sclerosis. *Practitioner* **192**, 540–542.

Bax, M., Goldstein, M., Rosenbaum, P., Leviton, A., Paneth, N., Dan, B., Jacobsson, B., Damiano, D. & Executive Committee for the Definition of Cerebral Palsy (2005): Proposed definition and classification of cerebral palsy, April 2005. *Dev. Med. Child Neurol.* **47**, 571–576.

Berg, M., Jahnsen, R., Froslie, K.F. & Hussain, A. (2004): Reliability of the Pediatric Evaluation of Disability Inventory (PEDI). *Phys. Occup. Ther Pediatr.* **24**, 61–77.

Bohannon, R.W. & Smith, M.B. (1987): Inter-rater reliability of a modified Ashworth scale of muscle spasticity. *Phys. Ther.* **67**, 206–207.

Boyce, F., Gowland, C., Rosenbaum, P.L, Lane, M., Plews, N., Goldsmith, C., et al. (1991): Measuring quality of movement in cerebral palsy: a review of instruments. *Phys. Ther.* **71**, 813–819.

Carswell, A., McColl, M.A., Baptiste, S., Law, M., Polatajko, H. & Pollock, N. (2004): The Canadian Occupational Performance Measure: a research and clinical literature review. *Can. J. Occup. Ther.* **71**, 210–222.

Charles, J., Wolf, S., Schneider, J. & Gordon, A. (2006): Efficacy of a child-friendly form of constraint-induced movement therapy in hemiplegic cerebral palsy: a randomized control trial. *Dev. Med. Child Neurol.* **48**, 635–642.

Cieza, A., Geyh, S., Chatterji, S., Kostanjsek, N., Ustund, B. & Stucki, G. (2005): ICF linking rules: an update based on lessons learned. *J. Rehabil. Med.* **37**, 212–218.

Cioni, G., Sgandurra, G., Muzzini, S., Paolicelli, P.B. & Ferrari, A. (2009): Forms of hemiplegia. In: *The Spastic Forms of Cerebral Palsy. A Guide to the Assessment of Adaptive Functions,* eds. A. Ferrari & G. Cioni, pp. 331–353. Milan: Springer-Verlag.

Coluccini, M., Maini, E.S., Martelloni, C., Sgandurra, G. & Cioni, G. (2007): Kinematic characterization of functional reach to grasp in normal and in motor disabled children. *Gait Posture* **25**, 493–501.

Cusick, A., Lannin, N.A. & Lowe, K. (2007): Adapting the Canadian Occupational Performance Measure for use in a paediatric clinical trial. *Disabil. Rehabil.* **29**, 761–766.

DeMatteo, C., Law, M., Russell, D.J., Pollock, N., Rosenbaum, P. & Walter, S. (1993): The reliability and validity of the Quality of Upper Extremity Skills Test. *Phys. Occup. Ther. Pediatr.* **13**, 1–18.

Eliasson, A.C. (2005): Normal and impaired development of force control in precision grip. In: *Hand Function in the Child: Foundation for Remediation*, eds. A. Henderson & C. Pehoski, pp. 45–61. New York: Elsevier–Mosby.

Eliasson, A.C., Gordon, A.M. & Forssberg, H. (1991): Basic co-ordination of manipulative forces of children with cerebral palsy. *Dev. Med. Child Neurol.* **33**, 661–670.

Eliasson, A.C., Krumlinde-Sundholm, L., Shaw, K. & Wang, C. (2005): Effects of constraint-induced movement therapy in young children with hemiplegic cerebral palsy: an adapted model. *Dev. Med. Child Neurol.* **47**, 266–275.

Eliasson, A.C., Forssberg, H., Hung, Y.C. & Gordon, A.M. (2006a): Development of hand function and precision grip control in individuals with cerebral palsy: a 13-year follow-up study. *Pediatrics* **118**, e1226–1236.

Eliasson, A.C., Krumlinde-Sundholm, L., Rösblad, B., Beckung, E., Arner, M., Öhrvall, A.M. & Rosenbaum, P. (2006b): Manual Ability Classification System (MACS) for children with cerebral palsy: scale development and evidence of validity and reliability. *Dev. Med. Child Neurol.* **48**, 549–554.

Eyre, J.A. (2003): Development and plasticity of the corticospinal system in man. *Neural Plast.* **10**, 93–106.

Eyre, J.A., Smith, M., Dabydeen, L., Clowry, G.J., Petacchi, E., Battini, R., *et al.* (2007): Is hemiplegic cerebral palsy equivalent to amblyopia of the corticospinal system? *Ann. Neurol.* **62**, 493–503.

Ferrari, A. & Cioni, G. (2005): *Le forme spastiche delle paralisi cerebrali infantili.* Milan: Springer-Verlag.

Forssberg, H., Eliasson, A.C., Kinoshita, H., Johansson, R.S. & Westling, G. (1991): Development of human precision grip. I: Basic coordination of force. *Exp. Brain Res.* **85**, 451–457.

Forssberg, H., Kinoshita, H., Eliasson, A.C., Johansson, R.S., Westling, G. & Gordon, A.M. (1992): Development of human precision grip. II: Anticipatory control of isometric forces targeted for object's weight. *Exp. Brain Res.* **90**, 393–398.

Fosang, A.L., Galea, M.P., McCoy, A.T., Reddihough, D.S. & Story, I. (2003): Measures of muscle and joint performance in the lower limb of children with cerebral palsy. *Dev. Med. Child Neurol.* **45**, 664–670.

Frye, R.E., Rotenberg, A., Ousley, M. & Pascual-Leone, M. (2008): Transcranial magnetic stimulation in child neurology: current and future directions. *J. Child Neurol.* **23**, 79–96.

Gilmore, R., Sakzewski, L. & Boyd, R. (2009): Upper limb activity measures for 5- to 16-year-old children with congenital hemiplegia: a systematic review. *Dev. Med. Child Neurol.* **52**, 14–21.

Gordon, A.M., Schneider, J.A., Chinnan, A. & Charles, J.R. (2007): Efficacy of a hand-arm bimanual intensive therapy (HABIT) in children with hemiplegic cerebral palsy: a randomized control trial. *Dev. Med. Child Neurol.* **49**, 830–838.

Guzzetta, A., Bonanni, P., Biagi, L., Tosetti, M., Montanaro, D., Guerrini, R. & Cioni, G. (2007): Reorganisation of the somatosensory system after early brain damage. *Clin. Neurophysiol.* **118**, 1110–1121.

Haga, N., van der Heijden-Maessen, H.C., van Hoorn, J.F., Boonstra, A.M. & Hadders-Algra, M. (2007): Test–retest and inter- and intra-reliability of the quality of the upper-extremity skills test in preschool-age children with cerebral palsy. *Arch. Phys. Med. Rehabil.* **88**, 1686–1689.

Haley, S.M., Coster, W.J., Ludlow, L.H., Haltiwanger, J.T. & Andrellos, P.J. (1992): *Pediatric Evaluation of Disability Inventory (PEDI): Development, Standardization and Administration manual.* Boston, MA: New England Medical Center.

Hanna, S., Russell, D., Bartlett, D., Kertoy, M., Rosenbaum, P. & Swinton, M. (2005): *Clinical measurement: Practical guidelines for service providers.* CanChild Centre for Childhood disability research. McMaster University.

Hoare, B.J., Wallen, M.A., Imms, C., Villanueva, E., Rawicki, H.B. & Carey, L. (2010). Botulinum toxin A as an adjunct to treatment in the management of the upper limb in children with spastic cerebral palsy (UPDATE) [review]. *Cochrane Database Syst. Rev.* **20,** CD003469.

Holmefur, M., Krumlinde-Sundholm, L. & Eliasson, A.C. (2007): Interrater and intrarater reliability of the Assisting Hand Assessment. *Am. J. Occup. Ther.* **61,** 79–84.

Holmstrom, L., Vollmer, B., Tedroff, K., Islam, M., Persson, J.K., Forssberg, H. & Eliasson, A.C. (2010): Hand function in relation to brain lesions and corticomotor-projection pattern in children with unilateral cerebral palsy. *Dev. Med. Child Neurol.* **52,** 145–152.

House, J.H., Gwathmey, F.W. & Fidler, M.O. (1981): A dynamic approach to the thumb-in-palm deformity in cerebral palsy: evaluation and results in fifty-six patients. *J. Bone Joint Surg.* **63(A),** 216–225.

Iyer, L.V., Haley, S.M., Watkins, M.P. & Dumans, H.M. (2003): Establishing minimal clinically important differences for scores on the pediatric evaluation of disability inventory for inpatient rehabilitation. *Phys. Ther.* **83,** 888–898.

Jebsen, R.H., Taylor, N., Trieschmann, R.B., Trotter, M.J. & Howard, L.A. (1969): An objective and standardised test of hand function. *Arch. Phys. Med. Rehabil.* **50,** 311–319.

Klingels, K., De Cock, P., Desloovere, K., Huenaerts, C., Molenaers, G., Van Nuland, I., et al. (2008): Comparison of the Melbourne Assessment of Unilateral Upper Limb Function and the Quality of Upper Extremity Skills Test in hemiplegic CP. *Dev. Med. Child Neurol.* **50,** 904–909.

Klingels, K., Jaspers, E., Van de Winckel, A., De Cock, P., Molenaers, G. & Feys, H. (2010): A systematic review of arm activity measures for children with hemiplegic cerebral palsy. *Clin. Rehabil.* **24,** 887–900.

Koman, L.A., Williams, R.M.M., Evans, P.J., Richardson, R., Naughton, M.J., Passmore, L. & Smith, B.P. (2008): Quantification of upper extremity function and range of motion in children with cerebral palsy. *Dev. Med. Child Neurol.* **50,** 910–917.

Krumlinde-Sundholm, L. (2008): Choosing and using assessment of hand function. In: *Improving Hand Function in Cerebral Palsy: Theory, Evidence and Intervention,* eds. A.C. Eliasson & P.A. Burtner, pp. 176–197. London: Mac Keith Press.

Krumlinde-Sundholm, L. & Eliasson, A.C. (2003): Development of the Assisting Hand Assessment: a Rasch-built measure intended for children with unilateral upper limb impairments. *Scand. J. Occup. Ther.* **10,** 16–26.

Krumlinde-Sundholm, L., Holmefur, M., Kottorp, A. & Eliasson, A.C. (2007): The Assisting Hand Assessment: current evidence of validity, reliability, and responsiveness to change. *Dev. Med. Child Neurol.* **49,** 259–264.

Law, M., Baptiste, S., Carswell, A., McColl, M.A., Polatajko, H. & Pollock, N. (1998): *Canadian occupational performance measure.* Ottawa: CAOT Publications.

Law, M., King, G., Russell, D., MacKinnon, E., Hurley, P. & Murphy, C. (1999): Measuring outcomes in children's rehabilitation: a decision protocol. *Arch. Phys. Med. Rehabil.* **80,** 629–636.

Morris, C., Kuriczuk, J.J., Fitzpatrick, R. & Rosenbaum, P. (2006): Reliability of the Manual Ability Classification System for children with cerebral palsy. *Dev. Med. Child Neurol.* **48,** 950–953.

Morris, S. (2002): Ashworth and Tardieu scales: their clinical relevance for measuring spasticity in adult and paediatric neurological populations. *Phys. Ther Rev.* **7,** 53–62.

Perazza, S., D'Avino, C. & Scapazzoni, P. (2008): Lesion and function: which relationship? Thesis, Master's degree in research in rehabilitation, University of Modena and Reggio Emilia.

Randall, M., Johnson, L. & Reddihough, D. (1999): *The Melbourne Assessment of Unilateral Upper Limb Function: Test administration manual.* Melbourne: Royal Children's Hospital.

Randall, M., Carlin, J.B., Chondros, P. & Reddihough, D. (2001): Reliability of the Melbourne Assessment of Unilateral Upper Limb Function. *Dev. Med. Child Neurol.* **43,** 761–767.

Randall, M., Imms, C. & Carey, L. (2008): Establishing validity of a modified Melbourne Assessment for children ages 2 to 4 years. *Am. J. Occup. Ther.* **62,** 373–383.

Rau, G., Disselhorst-Klug, C. & Schmidt, R. (2000): Movement biomechanics goes upwards: from the leg to the arm. *J. Biomech.* **33,** 1207–1216.

Rosenbaum, P. (1998). Screening tests and standardized assessments used to identify and characterize developmental delays. *Semin. Pediatr. Neurol.* **5,** 27–32.

Rosenbaum, P. & Stewart, D. (2004): The World Health Organization International Classification of Functioning, Disability, and Health: a model to guide clinical thinking, practice and research in the field of cerebral palsy. *Semin. Pediatr. Neurol.* **11,** 5–10.

Sakzewski, L., Boyd, R. & Ziviani, J. (2007): Clinimetric properties of participation measures for 5- to 13-year-old children with cerebral palsy: a systematic review. *Dev. Med. Child Neurol.* **49,** 232–240.

Sakzewski, L., Ziviani, J. & Boyd, R. (2010): The relationship between unimanual capacity and bimanual performance in children with congenital hemiplegia. *Dev. Med. Child Neurol.* **52,** 811–816.

Sorsdahl, A.B., Moe-Nilssen, R. & Strand, L.I. (2008): Observer reliability of the gross motor performance measure and the quality of upper extremity skills test, based on video recordings. *Dev. Med. Child Neurol.* **50,** 146–151.

Speth, L.A., Leffers, P., Janssen-Potten, Y.J. & Vles, J.S. (2005): Botulinum toxin A and upper limb functional skills in hemiparetic cerebral palsy: a randomised trial in children receiving intensive therapy. *Dev. Med. Child Neurol.* **47,** 468–473.

Steenbeek, D., Ketelaar, M., Linderman, E., Galama, K. & Gorter, J.W. (2010): Interrater reliability of goal attainment scaling in rehabilitation of children with cerebral palsy. *Arch. Phys. Med. Rehabil.* **91,** 429–435.

Taylor, N., Sand, P. & Jebsen, R. (1973): Evaluation of hand function in children. *Arch. Phys. Med. Rehabil.* **54,** 129–135.

Uvebrant, P. (1988): Hemiplegic cerebral palsy: aetiology and outcome. *Acta Paediatr. Scand.* **345,** 1–100.

Vargus-Adams, J. (2009): Understanding function and other outcomes in cerebral palsy. *Phys. Med. Rehabil. Clin. N. Am.* **20,** 567–575.

Wallen, M.A., O'Flaherty, S.J. & Waugh, M.C. (2004): Functional outcomes of intramuscular botulinum toxin type A in the upper limbs of children with cerebral palsy: a phase II trial. *Arch. Phys. Med. Rehabil.* **85,** 192–200.

Wallen, M.A., O'Flaherty, S.J. & Waugh, M.C. (2007): Functional outcomes of intra-muscular boutlinum toxin type A and occupational therapy in the upper limbs of children with cerebral palsy: a randomised controlled trial. *Arch. Phys. Med. Rehabil.* **88,** 1–10.

Wallen, M., Ziviani, J., Evans, R. & Novak, I. (2008): Modified constraint-induced therapy for children with hemiplegic cerebral palsy: a feasibility study. *Dev. Neurorehabil.* **11,** 124–133.

Waters, P.M., Zurakowski, D., Patterson, P. & Nimec, D. (2004): Interobserver and intraobserver reliability of therapist-assisted videotaped evaluations of upper-limb hemiplegia. *J. Hand. Surg.* **29(A),** 328–334.

Willis, J.K., Morello, A., Davie, A., Rice, J.C. & Bennett, J.T. (2002): Forced use treatment of childhood hemiparesis. *Pediatrics* **110,** 94–96.

World Health Organization (WHO) (2001): *The International Classification of Functioning, Disability and Health (ICF)*. Geneva: World Health Organization.

World Health Organization (2007): *International Classification of Functioning, Disability and Health–Children & Youth Version (ICF-CY)*. Geneva: World Health Organization.

Yam, W.K. & Leung, M.S. (2006): Interrater reliability of modified Ashworth Scale and modified Tardieu Scale in children with spastic cerebral palsy. *J. Child Neurol.* **21,** 1031–1035.

## Chapter 12

# Robotics and rehabilitation: new perspectives

Stefano Mazzoleni, Paolo Dario and Maria Chiara Carrozza

*The BioRobotics Institute, Scuola Superiore Sant'Anna,
Polo Sant'Anna Valdera, viale Rinaldo Piaggio 34,
56025 Pontedera, Pisa, Italy*
s.mazzoleni@sssup.it
dario@sssup.it
carrozza@sssup.it

## Summary

During the last decades, the potential of robotics as a tool for neuroscientific investigation has been demonstrated, thus contributing to increased knowledge of biological systems. On the other hand, a detailed analysis of the potentials of these systems (Dario *et al.*, 2003) based on recent neuroscientific achievements – particularly the mechanisms of neurogenesis and cerebral plasticity underlying motor learning and functional recovery after cerebral injury – highlights the advisability of using robotic technologies, as systems able to contribute to a breakthrough in clinical neurorehabilitative treatments. Several examples of robotic machines applied to both neuroscience and neurorehabilitation can be found in the literature (Colombo *et al.*, 2000; Krebs *et al.*, 1998). One of the main scientific and technological challenges is represented by the design and development of innovative robotic and mechatronic systems able to (i) simplify interactive modalities during assisted motor exercises, (ii) enhance adaptability of the machines to the patient's performance and residual abilities, and (iii) provide a comprehensive picture of the psycho-physiological status of the patient for assessment purposes through the integrated use of brain imaging techniques.

The basic assumption of this work relies on a human-centred approach applied to the design of robotic and mechatronic devices aimed at carrying out neuroscientific investigations of human sensorimotor behaviour, delivering innovative neurorehabilitation therapies, and assessing the functional recovery of disabled patients. Special attention is paid to the issues related to human–machine interactivity adapted to human motor mechanisms and the design of machines for the analysis of human motor behaviour and the quantitative assessment of motor performance.

## Introduction

In industrialized societies, several factors contribute to a growing need for rehabilitative services as complement and support to surgical and pharmacologic treatments. The major factor is (*a*) the increasing longevity of the population, to which is added (*b*) the reduction in the duration of hospitalization, (*c*) the use of therapies that can treat highly progressive debilitating diseases, (*d*) the increased incidence of severe and moderate disabilities resulting from activities that risk injury and trauma, and (*e*) the use of advanced techniques of resuscitation.

The need for appropriate rehabilitative therapies is increasingly important in many motor disorders of neurologic origin: in this case, we refer more specifically to *neurorehabilitation*.

Millions of people worldwide suffer from motor disorders associated with neurologic problems such as stroke, brain and spinal cord injuries, multiple sclerosis, and Parkinson disease.

A brief look at the situation in Italy shows the impact of these diseases: each year in Italy about 196,000 strokes occur[1] in which approximately 20 per cent of those affected die within the first month after the acute event and another 30 per cent of survivors are severely disabled. Of these 196,000 strokes, 80 per cent are first episodes, whereas 20 per cent are relapses.

Stroke represents the third leading cause of death in industrialized countries, after cardiovascular disease and cancer, and it is the leading cause of disability, exerting a significant impact at the individual, family, and social levels (Feigin *et al.*, 2003; Marini *et al.*, 2004; Murray *et al.*, 1997).

The incidence of stroke progressively increases with age, reaching its maximum in persons over 85 years old (24.2 per cent), with a predominance of male (28.2 per cent) over female (21.8 per cent) incidence. The prevalence of stroke in the Italian elderly population (age 65–84 years) is equivalent to 6.5 per cent and is slightly higher in men (7.4 per cent) than in women (5.9 per cent). Stroke affects young people, although to a lesser extent: every year about 25.0 per cent of the stroke episodes affects people of productive age (< 65 years) (SPREAD, 2010).

In the US, the estimated cost of hospitalization due to stroke in 1998 is $68.9 billion (Heart Disease and Stroke Statistics 2009 Update).

Traditional methods of therapy present some limitations, which are important to note. In many of the above-mentioned cases, the traditional motor rehabilitative approaches involve manipulation of the paretic upper limb by the therapist. Usually the treatment is planned by assessing the residual abilities of the subject *ex ante* and can last several hours a day: it can be often a long and exhausting exercise for both the patient and the therapist.

Therapeutic treatments can be extended for several months after hospitalization, during which patients must travel daily to the clinical facilities, posing severe hardship on themselves and their family. Moreover, for many motor disorders the therapeutic approaches and clinical protocols that are objectively more effective for a better recovery of motor function are not yet sufficiently clear, partly because the residual abilities of the patient are often assessed by using largely subjective measurements, thus making it difficult to adequately evaluate the effects of the therapeutic rehabilitation on the patient.

The nature of these treatments, which have to be administered by therapists one patient at a time, and the lack of methodologies and tools able to compare the different rehabilitative therapies and their effectiveness, make the costs associated with rehabilitation services typically high; thus, the ratio between the number of qualified human personnel available for rehabilitative services and the number of patients requiring them is often higher than one. It is also difficult to define methods for assessing and improving the cost/effectiveness ratio related to specific rehabilitation programs.

---

[1] Data extrapolated from the population in 2001.

The use of robotic machines for neurorehabilitation is inspired by neurophysiologic evidence showing that, starting from the cellular level, synaptic connections undergo continuous changes in response to physiologic events, environmental stimuli (processes of learning and memory), and damage to the central nervous system (CNS)[2].

The topology of the motor and sensory cortex is not fixed, but rather is flexible and adaptable to learning and experience (Donoghue *et al.*, 1996). This characteristic of the motor cortex has important implications for rehabilitation: (*a*) rapid changes in cortical activity can occur; (*b*) the intensive training of the cortical area may occur at the surrounding areas' expense; and (*c*) cortical areas can adapt their functions to those changes.

Thanks to such brain imaging techniques as functional magnetic resonance imaging (fMRI), positron emission tomography (PET), transcranial magnetic stimulation (TMS) associated with motor evoked potentials (MEPs) and electrical stimulation, changes in the CNS's excitability and topology can be shown. Through the use of such techniques, it is possible to identify regions that have suffered damage and to apply a specific therapy.

Sensorimotor learning is influenced by physical (sensory feedback such as vision, hearing, and proprioception), psychological (pleasure/pain, motivation, emotional impulses, and desire), and cognitive (decision making, planning, reasoning, concentration and attention, language and understanding, previous experiences) factors.

Sensorimotor learning can be facilitated by the repetition of movements directed to specific targets (goal-oriented movements), the strengthening of muscles and the increase of the range of motion (ROM), the modulation of spasticity, an increased demand for focusing attention on movement, and the increase of sensory stimuli.

In recent years different research groups have studied and developed innovative robotic and mechatronic systems able to let the patient perform repetitive and goal-oriented movements. These systems can provide a safe and intensive training[3] that can be carried out in association with other types of treatment, appropriate to different residual motor abilities, and that are potentially able to significantly improve the rehabilitation outcomes, to make an objective assessment, and to improve the planning and use of healthcare resources.

In rehabilitation assisted by a robot, the patient's role is undoubtedly central: the machine supports, and, if necessary, completes, the movement performed by the patient according to his/her residual motor abilities ('assisted as needed' control strategy).

Persons suffering from motor disorders can perform rehabilitation therapy with the support of a 'rehabilitation machine'[4].

---

[2] The terms *neuroplasticity* or *neural plasticity* are used to point out the sequence of changes in chemical (interaction between neurotransmitter and receptor), electrical (long-term depression and long-term potentiation), and molecular (activation of transcription factors and protein synthesis) responses, which lead to a reorganization of connections in the cerebral areas and, consequently, to cognitive changes and stable behaviours.

[3] During each training session using robotic systems, a high number of movements can be performed: the repetition of motor actions is a factor which can promote the recovery of motor functions.

[4] A 'rehabilitation machine' is a mechatronic or robotic system able to support the therapist during the administration of programmable and customized rehabilitation programs. It is composed of a mechanical structure where the following modules are present: (1) actuators; (2) energy supply; (3) proprioceptive and exteroceptive sensors, providing information on the machine's status and the interaction between the machine and the environment, respectively; (4) a microcontroller, dedicated to the processing of data from sensors and generation of motor control commands; and (5) a human–machine interface (graphical user interface) dedicated to user inputs, data recording, and feedback output.

The patient, through interaction with these systems receives different sensorimotor and cognitive inputs, such as proprioceptive and visual *stimuli* and motivational incentives[5]: by using appropriate sensors, the machine is capable of measuring dynamic variables of clinical interest during the performance of active and passive movements by the patient. Thus, a quantitative assessment of specific physiologic mechanisms and of motor recovery and functional skills can be carried out. This type of assessment is much more accurate than those using traditional methods. In addition, the machine may enable the therapist to plan the treatment and let the patient execute a wide sequence of movements, which can be useful for limb rehabilitation.

The application of machines to rehabilitation is sometimes limited by technical and functional factors; their real advantage in clinical applications has been only partially proved. However, there are solid arguments that encourage researchers to design and develop innovative systems for rehabilitation which derive a direct benefit from the scientific and technological progress in the field of bioengineering, particularly in biomedical robotics and mechatronics.

The clinical potential of these machines, however, is clearly significant, as they can, on the one hand, assist the therapist in the administration of a patient-specific physical therapy, with the accuracy and repeatability typical of robotic systems, and on the other hand, they can acquire quantitative information on the patient's movements.

Such information may be useful for the evaluation of both the patient's motor function and the mechanisms of motor recovery. These machines can also enable the patient to perform rehabilitative sessions in a semi-autonomous modality, and, in principle, even at his/her own home, thus reducing the need for the therapist's continuous commitment[6].

The technological innovation in robotics and mechatronics that has already been achieved has shown encouraging results in the knowledge of motor recovery mechanisms and contributed to real progress in the rehabilitation field that has a potential high impact.

In the wide range of technological applications developed in the context of biomedical robotics, undoubtedly a class of particular importance is represented by the systems for the rehabilitation of patients who have reduced mobility after an injury or disease.

In the next paragraphs, robotic systems for patients with the need for upper and lower extremity rehabilitation will be discussed including mechatronic systems for functional assessment as well as movement analysis.

## Robotic systems for upper limb rehabilitation

The World Health Organization (WHO, 2004) estimates that each year 15 million people worldwide are affected by a stroke and 5 million of those are living with a permanent disability. The majority of post-stroke patients are able to recover independent walking, but many of them fail to obtain a functional use of upper limbs even after prolonged rehabilitation: these functional limitations are responsible for a significant reduction in quality of life (Nichols-Larsen *et al.*, 2005).

---

[5] The patient often feels rewarded by the use of high-tech systems for rehabilitation. Besides, motivational incentives are strongly stimulated by the use of graphical interfaces which provide a feedback on the performed movements, which are linked to the recovery of essential functionalities for his/her daily life.

[6] This therapy, known as 'tele-rehabilitation', is based on the integration of high-tech systems (*e.g.*, a robotic system for rehabilitation) and telecommunication infrastructures (*e.g.*, cable connections, optical fibres, wireless networks, and satellite systems): it is aimed at enabling the execution of rehabilitation treatments at the patient's own home or rehabilitation centre through the direct remote supervision and monitoring by physicians and therapists.

One year after the acute event, the condition of the patients is usually considered chronic, and rehabilitative therapies are often suspended (Duncan *et al.*, 1992); several studies have shown that improvements in motor abilities induced by rehabilitative therapies may also occur in patients with chronic damage from 6 to 12 months after the acute event (Hendricks *et al.*, 2002). Recent approaches that involve repetitive training of the upper limbs with activities aimed at task-oriented movements have provided evidence of improvements in hemiparetic patients more than a year after the stroke. In particular, constraint-induced movement therapy (CIMT), based on an intense practice functionally oriented to hemiparetic upper limb tasks obtained by a restriction of the unimpaired upper limb seems to be effective in reducing long-term disability (Miltner *et al.*, 1999; Wolf *et al.*, 2006). The motivation for using this type of treatment is based on the evidence that stroke and other neurologic damage cause a partial destruction of cortical tissue, with the involvement of sensorimotor areas that can determine incorrect motor programmes. However, CIMT requires a significant level of motor function and is not suitable for patients with severe weakness or spasticity due to neurologic damage.

Other treatments based on high-intensity and task-oriented active upper limb movements led to significant improvements in cortical reorganization and motor function in people with disabilities more than a year after the stroke (Fasoli *et al.*, 2008). Unfortunately, these traditional treatments for post-stroke rehabilitation show some drawbacks: they require manual interaction with the therapists that must be provided on a daily basis for several weeks: the administration of an intensive treatment for each patient is difficult and costly.

Several robotic devices for rehabilitation have been recently developed to overcome these disadvantages: they are able to provide a safe and intensive therapy to patients with different degrees of motor impairment (Riener *et al.*, 2005a). Furthermore, the training with the support of the robot can be extremely precise, intense, and prolonged. The robotic systems can also measure the progress of the patient in an objective way, increasing the effectiveness of treatment and reducing the costs associated with the healthcare system.

Several reviews have shown the robot-assisted sensorimotor treatments and task-oriented repetitive movements can improve muscle strength and motor coordination in patients with neurologic damage (Kwakkel *et al.*, 2008; Mehrholz *et al.*, 2008), although a limited number of clinical studies have examined the effect of upper limb robot-aided post-stroke rehabilitation using robust study designs (*i.e.*, randomized controlled trial)[7].

Among these, only three studies involved more than 30 subjects, and only two trials focused on pre- and post-treatment measures in experimental and control groups (Lum *et al.*, 2002; Krebs *et al.*, 2000), of which only one was an RCT about the effects of the robot therapy provided to patients in the subacute phase (Krebs *et al.*, 2000).

Among the most advanced robotic systems providing a growing amount of experimental data, the 'MIT-Manus' (InMotion[2], Interactive Motion Technologies. Inc., Cambridge, MA, USA), designed at the Massachusetts Institute of Technology (MIT), holds a special role (Hogan *et al.*, 1995) (Fig. 1a). The clinical trial was started in 1994 at the Burke Rehabilitation Hospital (White Plains, NY, USA) and recently many hospitals around the world use the MIT-Manus robotic system as a tool for upper extremity rehabilitation therapy in patients with neurologic damage.

---

[7] A randomized controlled trial (RCT) represents the most rigorous way of determining the cause–effect relation between treatment and outcome. It is a study in which recruited participants are randomly allocated to receive one of several clinical interventions. One of these interventions is the control (*e.g.*, a standard practice), the other is the experimental treatment (*e.g.*, robot-aided therapy).

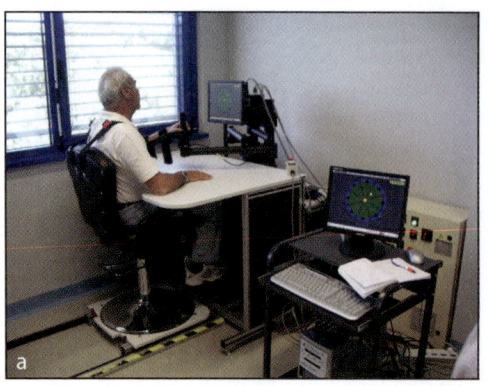 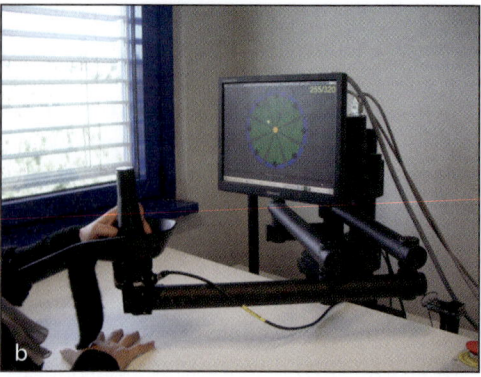

*Fig. 1. A patient during the MIT-Manus robotic therapy (**a**) and end-effector of the robotic system (**b**).*

In Europe, the first example of this robotic system was purchased by the Scuola Superiore Sant'Anna in Pisa, Italy in 2005 and is currently at the Neurological Rehabilitation and Traumatic Brain Injury Unit at Rehabilitation Centre 'Auxilium Vitae' in Volterra, Italy, where clinical trials on hemiparetic subjects are in progress.

The MIT-Manus system is an operational-type robotic device characterized by a human–machine interface which is limited to the robot's end-effector[8] (Fig. 1b). Unlike the case in industrial robots, where any contact with the human operator is usually excluded for safety reasons, the MIT-Manus was specifically designed to interact with the patient in a safe, stable, and, when necessary, compliant way.

These characteristics are obtained through the use of a control scheme, called 'impedance control', which modulates the movement of the robot in order to adapt itself to the patient's upper limb dynamics. The MIT-Manus can move, drive, or disturb the upper movement of a subject and enables the recording of significant variables such as position, speed, and the forces applied at the end-effector (Krebs *et al.*, 1998). The distinctive characteristics of the MIT-Manus robotic system are a high reversibility mechanism (back-drivability) and a low mechanical impedance, which can readily adapt to the actions of the patient, and the control system, which through the above-mentioned 'impedance control' modulates the reactions of the system to mechanical disturbances and ensures compliant behaviour[9].

In fact, the machine was designed so as to have an intrinsic low impedance, low isotropic inertia (0:33 ± 1 kg; maximum anisotropy 2:1), low isotropic friction (0:28 ± 0.84 N; maximum anisotropy 2:1) and is capable of producing a definite range of forces (0–45 N) and impedance (0–2 N/mm).

The rehabilitation treatment using the MIT-Manus consists of a series of complex motor tasks to be performed by the patient, who is asked to move the robot's end-effector (Fig. 1a) to perform movements aimed at hitting targets in a bidimensional space (reaching tasks). Specific biomechanical parameters, which are computed starting from the above-mentioned physical variables recorded by the MIT-Manus system, can be used for the characterization of the patient's motor performance, together with other parameters calculated from the electroencephalographic signals (EEG) for the assessment of motor area activation, before and after treatment (Fig. 2).

---

[8] A different class of robotic systems for rehabilitation is represented by the exoskeleton-type systems, where the contact between the patient and the machine is extended to the whole impaired limb (or part of it).

[9] The robot assists the patient's movements in order to make their execution easier: only if the patient is not able to perform a movement does the robot's control system assist and guide the paretic upper limb in order to complete it.

Chapter 12  Robotics and rehabilitation: new perspectives

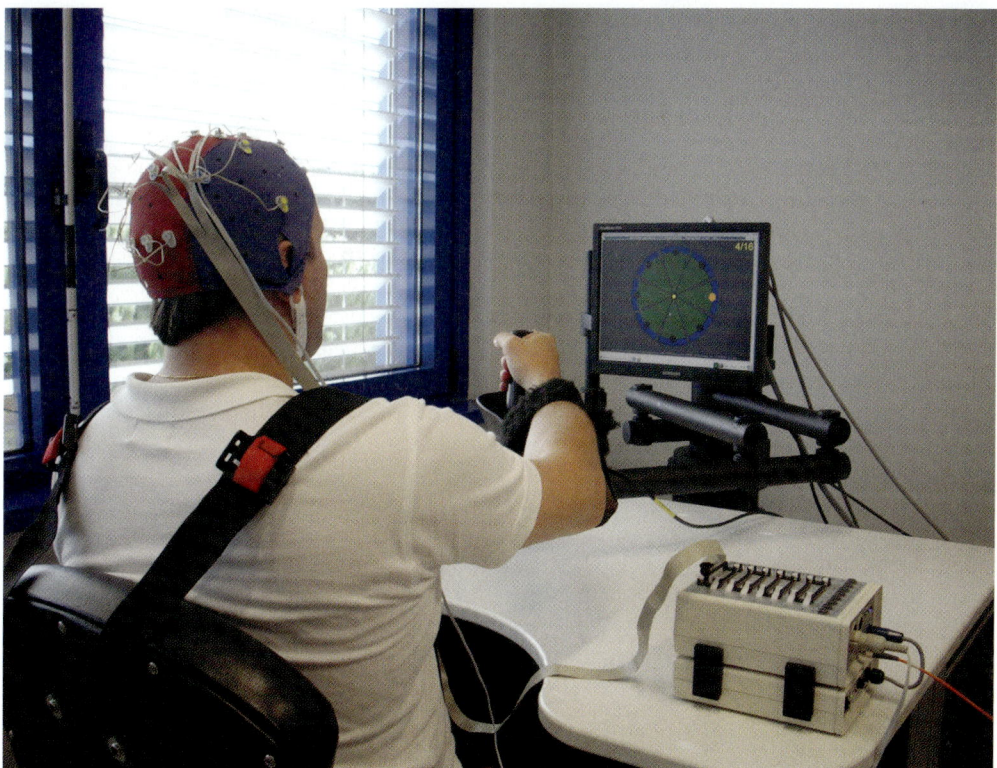

Fig. 2. A subject during the robotic therapy using the MIT-Manus and recording EEG signals for the functional assessment.

The different clinical experimental trials performed using MIT-Manus were described in several articles (Fasoli *et al.*, 2003, 2004; Ferraro *et al.*, 2003; Volpe *et al.*, 1999). The results of a study performed on 96 patients, including 40 subjects in the control group and 56 subjects in the experimental group, showed an improvement of the latter over the former according to the results of functional assessment performed by using different clinical scales, including the motor status score for the shoulder and elbow (MSS-SE), the motor power scale (MP), and the modified Ashworth scale (MAS) (Volpe *et al.*, 2000).

The results of our clinical trials confirm the significant improvement of motor damage by (1) an increase in MSS-SE values for both the shoulder and the elbow joint, (2) a decrease in the MAS values for the shoulder joint, (3) no increase in the MAS values for the elbow joint, and (4) an increase of the ROM for the shoulder joint: the data are statistically significant and were recorded before and after treatment in chronic hemiparetic subjects: the treatment was administered for 6 weeks (three sessions per week at 45 minutes for each session) (Posteraro *et al.*, 2009, 2010).

The 3 months' follow-up study has revealed a further reduction of the motor damage due to an increase in the ROM of the shoulder joint.

In conclusion, our results showed that the improvement in motor skills after neurologic damage may continue even a year after the acute event.

The results of the questionnaires designed to measure the acceptability of the robotic therapy, which were distributed to the patients at the end of the experimental trial, showed a substantial acceptance of the robotic therapy, which, however, cannot be considered as a substitute for the traditional rehabilitation treatments and the role of the therapist.

A clinical trial currently in progress with hemiparetic subjects in the subacute phase is aimed at assessing the effects of robotic therapy a few weeks after the acute event and identifying prognostic parameters of motor recovery to be provided to physiatrists in order to identify early the most suitable rehabilitative treatments for each patient.

Another robotic system for the upper limb rehabilitation of post-stroke patients, the 'MEMOS' (mechatronic system for motor recovery after stroke), was designed and developed at the Scuola Superiore Sant'Anna in Pisa, Italy (Fig. 3). It is currently used at the Fondazione Salvatore Maugeri in Veruno, Italy, where clinical trials have already shown excellent results: a significant reduction of upper limb impairment in chronic hemiparetic patients was observed (Micera *et al.*, 2005; Colombo *et al.*, 2005, 2008).

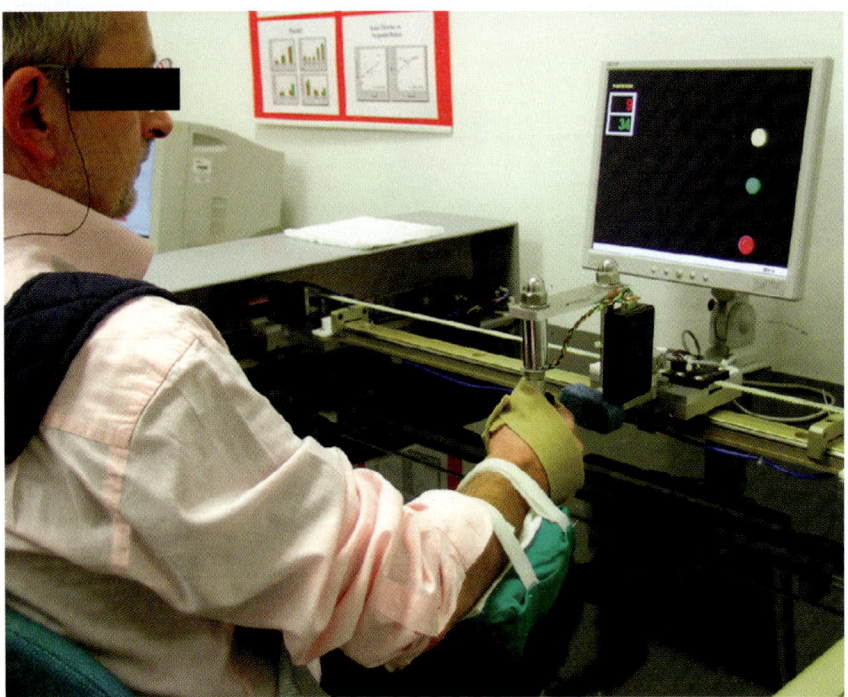

*Fig. 3. The MEMOS system: a mechatronic system for upper limb rehabilitation.*

The MEMOS enables patients to perform reaching movements using a simple system of mechanical guides: the dimensions of its workspace are 70 cm × 70 cm. Before the therapy session is started, the worktable can be tilted by the therapist according to the needs of the patient by means of manual adjustment. Adding greater simplicity in terms of mechanical structure compared to the MIT-Manus, the MEMOS adds the flexibility of a system that can be used for rehabilitation at home, supported in real-time by the remote control of physiatrists and therapists.

## Robotic systems for lower limb rehabilitation

The objective of rehabilitation in paraplegic patients is to achieve maximum independence in the activities of daily living (ADL). Over the past decades, the rehabilitation of locomotion in individuals with spinal cord injury (SCI) was largely developed and tested (Barbeau & Rossignol, 1994; Barbeau et al., 1999, 2006; Scivoletto & Di Donna, 2009). Currently, the locomotion in these subjects is performed using standard wheelchairs, often without any training for the functional motor recovery of the lower limbs (i.e., the gait).

Increasing evidence based on neurophysiologic studies has demonstrated the ability to activate locomotion patterns in animals affected by a spinal cord injury through the use of systems for body weight support (BWS) and a treadmill (Barbeau & Rossignol, 1987). Similar studies were performed on human subjects using a harness and variable BWS percentages on the treadmill: the locomotion activities in SCI subjects can be improved using such systems (Dietz & Colombo, 2004; Edgerton et al., 2006; Grasso et al., 2004; Scivoletto et al., 2007).

To activate the locomotor function using this approach, it is often necessary to help the progression of the lower limbs on a treadmill through the manual effort of two or more therapists. Therefore the duration of the training is usually limited by the fatigue of the therapists, which results in a shorter duration of the sessions than that needed to obtain a good rehabilitative outcome. To facilitate this type of rehabilitation and to ensure repeatability of the movements for locomotion, the 'Lokomat' system (Hocoma AG, Volketswil, Switzerland), a bilateral robotic orthosis used in conjunction with a BWS system and a treadmill, has been developed (Fig. 4) (Colombo et al., 2000, 2001).

The joints in the Lokomat system, located in correspondence to the hip and knee joint, are moved by linear actuators which are integrated into the exoskeletal structure. A passive system of springs aimed at lifting the foot's sole induces the ankle's dorsiflexion during the swing phase. The patient's lower limbs, which are fixed to the exoskeletal structure through adjustable straps and settings, are moved in the *sagittal* plane according to a control strategy with predefined hip and knee trajectories, which enables a safe patient-machine interaction (Riener et al., 2005b; Riener et al., 2006). Various studies have been published about the use of the Lokomat system in subjects affected by neurologic diseases (Colombo et al., 2000; Hidler & Wall, 2005; Hidler et al., 2009; Hornby et al., 2008; Israel et al., 2006; Jezernik et al., 2003; Lünenburger et al., 2005, 2006; Wirz et al., 2005).

Recent experimental studies analyzed the activation of different EMG patterns in healthy and spinal cord-injured (SCI) subjects during the Lokomat training using the treadmill in different experimental conditions (Hidler & Wall, 2005). The comparison of the EMG activity between healthy and SCI subjects shows that in a complete spinal cord injury, the adaptation to different speeds is still present (Lünenberger et al., 2006).

An experimental collaborative study currently in progress, carried out by the Scuola Superiore Sant'Anna and the Neurorehabilitation Unit and the Spinal Cord Injuries Departmental Unit at Cisanello Hospital in Pisa, is aimed at assessing the changes in muscle activation after a period of rehabilitation using the Lokomat system in subjects with incomplete spinal cord injury.

To our current knowledge, the use of this device is still experimental; the choice of the variable parameters (BWS percentage, speed, driving force, and duration) is not yet included in specific guidelines, and the patterns of muscular activation of the robot-aided gait are not, for the time being, well defined.

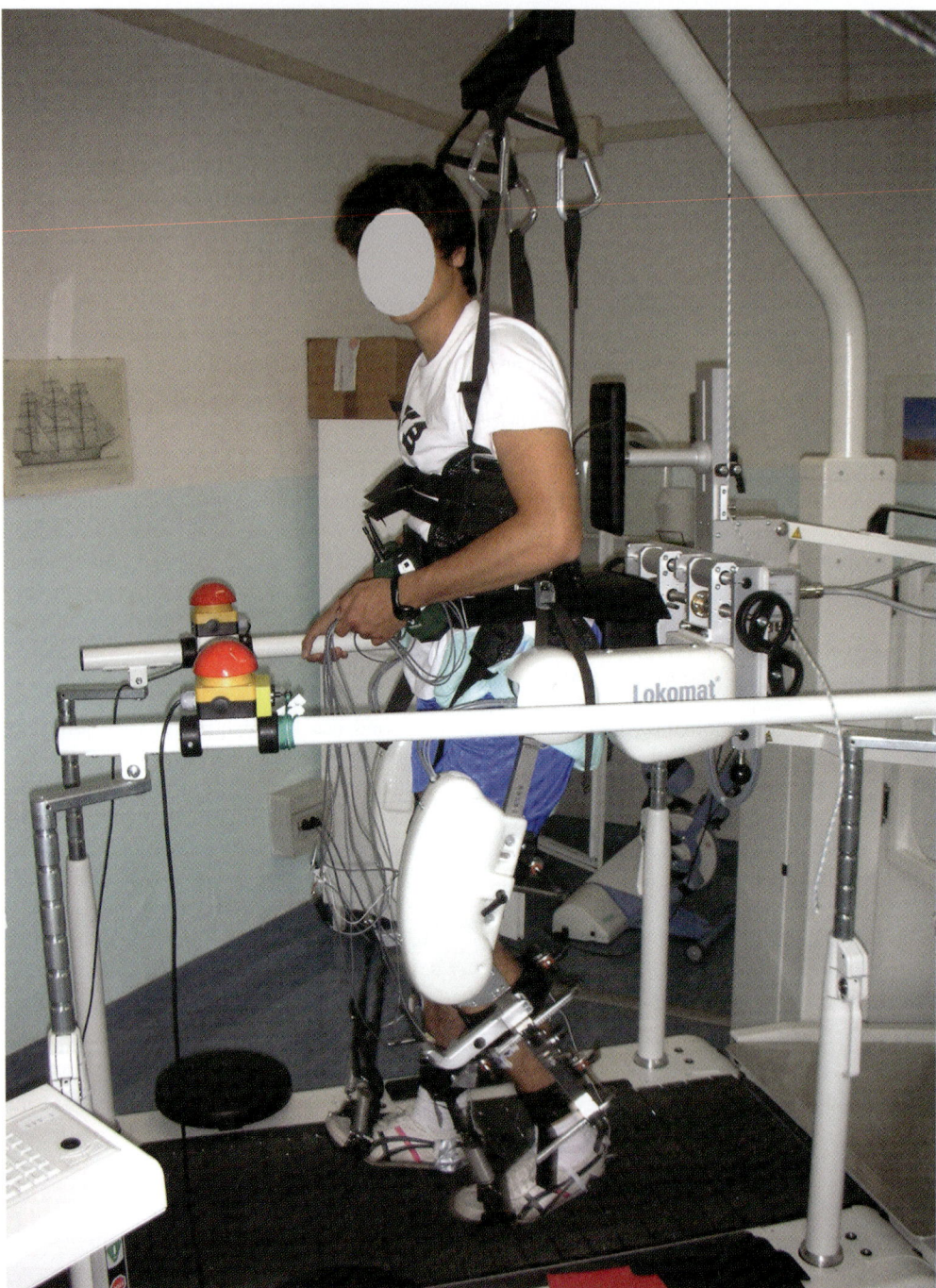

Fig. 4. The Lokomat robotic system for lower limb rehabilitation.

Surface EMG signals from four muscles on each limb (rectus femoris, biceps femoris, anterior tibial, and medial gastrocnemius) in healthy subjects and in patients with incomplete spinal cord injury during the training with the Lokomat robotic system have been recorded. In detail, three different treadmill speeds (1.0, 1.6, and 2.4 km/h) using two BWS percentages (30 per cent and 60 per cent) and two different patient cooperation modalities were used. These modalities are: (1) *passive*, in which the subject does not contribute to the movement of the lower limbs that are mobilized by the robotic orthosis, and (2) *active*, in which the subject accompanies the movement of the lower limbs according to his or her residual motor abilities.

Subjects with a spinal cord injury follow, after a first recording (pre-training), a training program with the Lokomat system of variable duration (*i.e.*, 4–8 weeks), after which a further EMG recording is performed (post-training). Follow-up recordings at 3 and 6 months are performed as well.

So far, the results obtained on a limited sample of patients with incomplete spinal cord injury undergoing physical therapy using the Lokomat robotic system showed an improvement of the locomotor function because of enhanced recruitment of the lower limb muscles in the 'active' condition: the assessment was based on the analysis of EMG signals recorded before and after the treatment, using specific clinical scales (*i.e.*, 10-meter walk test, 6-minute walk test, timed 'up & go' test) (Mazzoleni *et al.*, 2008).

## Mechatronic systems for functional assessment and movement analysis

*Mechatronics* is defined as the synergistic integration of mechanical engineering, with electronics and intelligent computer control, in the design and manufacture of industrial products and processes (Harashima *et al.*, 1996). A mechatronic approach has several benefits. In fact, mechatronic systems have greater flexibility, a better performance, higher quality, wide areas of applications, and are less expensive.

Here we focus on the applications of mechatronics to the rehabilitation with respect to two main research fields: functional assessment and movement analysis.

A mechatronic platform for the functional assessment of the rehabilitation treatment using isometric force/torque during the execution of ADL tasks in post-stroke subjects was designed and developed within the ALLADIN project, funded by the European Commission under the 6th Framework Program (IST-2002-507424) (<www.alladin-ehealth.org>).

The platform (Fig. 5) was validated in three clinical centers in Europe: (1) Mary Middelares Algemeen Ziekenhuis Sint-Jozef (Gent, Belgium); (2) Szent János Hospital (Budapest, Hungary); and (3) Adelaide & Meath Hospital (Tallaght, Co. Dublin, Ireland).

In these centres, an experimental clinical trial with 270 subjects (150 hemiparetic subjects and 120 healthy control subjects) was carried out: the results identified six parameters related to the motor recovery of post-stroke patients that can be used to perform a functional assessment a short time after the acute event so that physiatrists and therapists can quickly choose the most appropriate rehabilitative treatment for each patient (Mazzoleni *et al.*, 2009).

In recent years, different wearable mechatronic systems for movement analysis were developed. The MEKA (MEchatronic device for Knee Analysis) system, collaboratively designed and developed by the ARTS Lab at Scuola Superiore Sant'Anna in Pisa, Italy and Humanware, Inc., (Pisa, Italy) is a mechatronic device that performs a real-time monitoring of the knee's flexion-extension and varus-valgus angles (knee's dynamic analysis) during the gait and other ADL. The recorded data can be displayed in a numeric and graphic format.

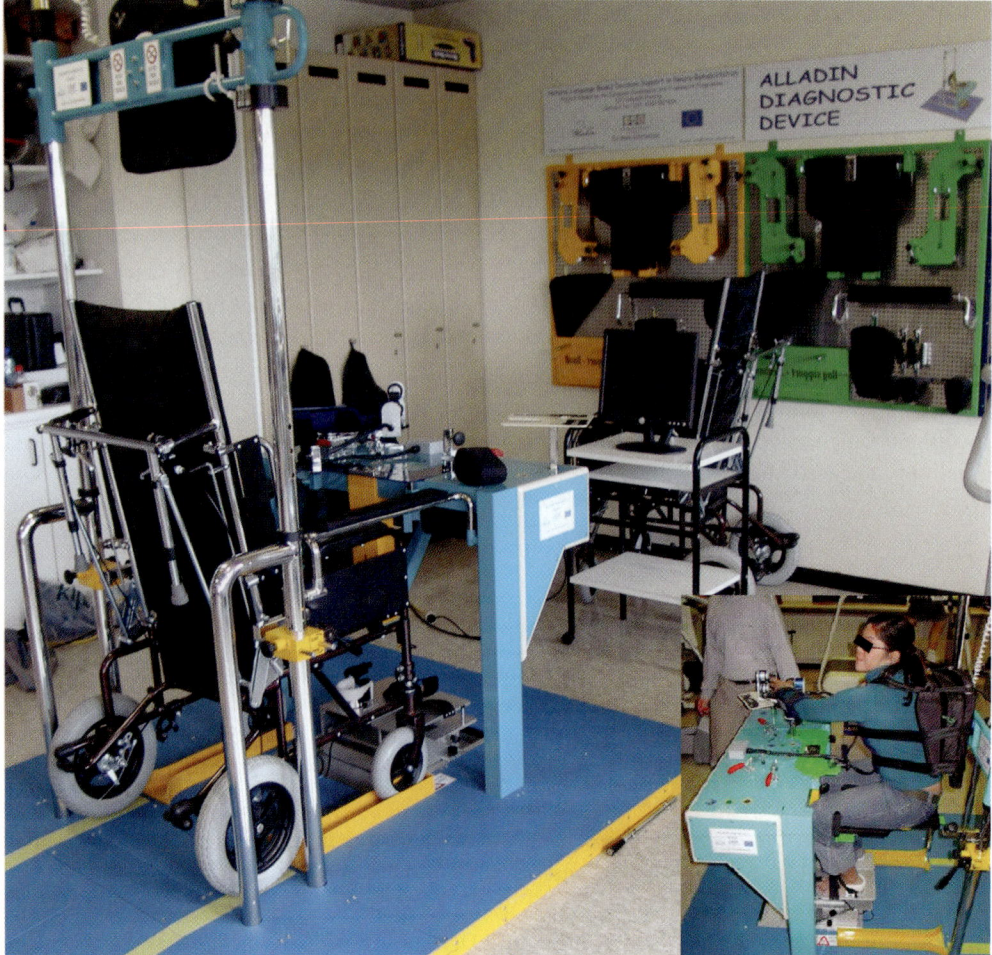

*Fig. 5. The ALLADIN mechatronic platform for functional assessment of post-stroke subjects.*

The system is composed of three main units:

(1) a modular mechatronic device for measuring values from the knee's flexion–extension and varus–valgus angles through the use of Hall-effect sensors (Fig. 6a);
(2) a wireless system for the kinematic data acquisition and transfer to PC (Fig. 6b); and
(3) a software tool for processing and displaying data.

One of the main advantages of the MEKA system is the best cost/effectiveness ratio when compared to similar devices aimed at performing a similar knee's dynamic analysis.

The results of experiments carried out by using such a mechatronic device highlighted different locomotor strategies, depending on the age and the difficulty of the required task (Micera *et al.*, 2003, 2004).

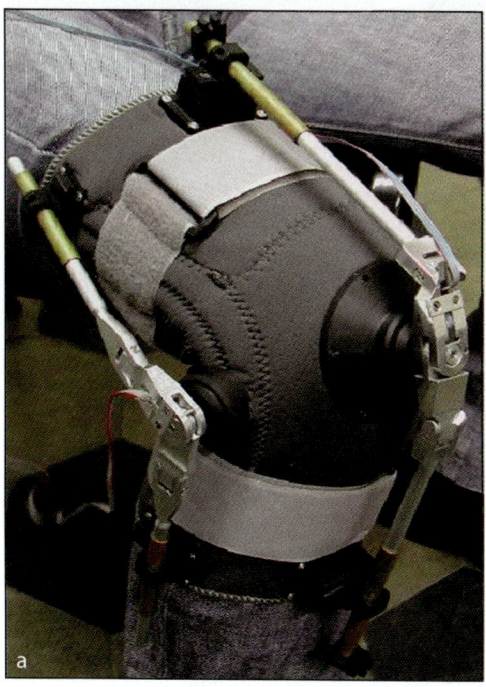 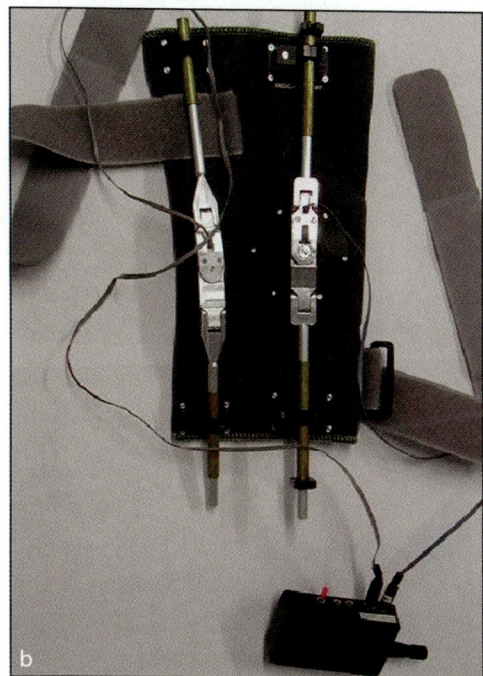

Fig. 6. *The MEKA mechatronic system for knee-movement analysis.*

## Applications of robotic and mechatronic technologies to paediatric rehabilitation

Recent results show that paediatric subjects affected by cerebral palsy improve gait parameters after rehabilitation training by means of a robotic system assisting mobilization of the lower limbs (Borggraefe *et al.*, 2010; Meyer-Heim *et al.*, 2009) (Fig. 7, *left*).

The same robotic device was used in a rehabilitation programme in combination with a virtual reality system. Children have shown a positive feedback for such rehabilitation treatment, in terms of motivation and participation (Koenig *et al.*, 2008).

The use of robotic systems for upper limb rehabilitation (Fig. 7, *right*) can be considered an effective tool to be included in the rehabilitation programme for paediatric hemiparetic patients (Petrarca *et al.*, 2009). Recent studies have demonstrated that the introduction of robotic systems in the rehabilitation of paediatric patients with neurologic disease can contribute to the recovery of motor function (Borggraefe *et al.* 2008; Frascarelli *et al.*, 2009; Meyer-Heim *et al.*, 2007), which was affirmed by the patients' perception of the recovery of the limb's functional use at home (Fasoli *et al.*, 2008). Thus we see that using robotic systems for rehabilitation in children has an additional advantage in terms of motivation and participation of these patients in the training activities.

Studies with larger populations and multicenter randomized controlled trials (RCTs) are necessary to confirm the encouraging results obtained so far and to evaluate in depth both the effectiveness of robot-assisted treatments for the rehabilitation of paediatric patients and its efficacy for national healthcare systems as assessed by specific Healthcare Technology Assessment (HTA) procedures.

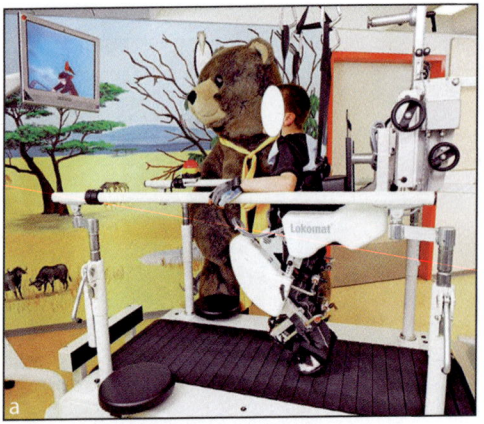 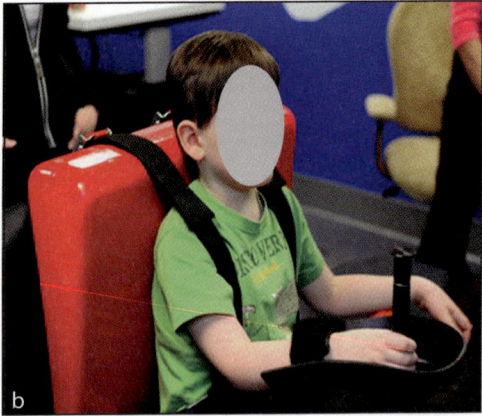

*Fig. 7. Robotic systems for rehabilitation of neurologic disease in paediatric patients.*

## Open issues

In the field of robotics and mechatronic systems for rehabilitation some problems are still unsolved, requiring further development. In terms of clinical trials, the main issues are:

– the need for a greater number of patients to be recruited in clinical trials;
– the use of homogeneous groups of patients and control groups (*i.e.*, a randomized clinical trial);
– the development of innovative clinical protocols;
– the definition of quantitative parameters related to the rehabilitation treatment (milestones) and prognostic parameters (markers);
– the identification of neurophysiologic models of the recovery process;
– the detailed analysis of scenarios and definition of the roles of involved subjects (patient, physiatrist, and therapist); and
– the incremental innovation of devices already available and the design of new technological systems for rehabilitation.

A key requirement concerns the active role that the patient has to take during the administration of robotic therapy: the patient's ability to participate actively should be taken into account when designing new technological systems for rehabilitation. Furthermore, the integration between robotic systems and the techniques of brain imaging for functional evaluation represents a fundamental area of research in order to define therapeutic approaches tailored to the specific needs of each patient and the degree of recovery.

## Conclusions

The robotic and mechatronic systems presented in this chapter are increasingly used in hospitals and rehabilitation centres as technological tools for clinical practice. These systems are used to administer intensive and prolonged treatments aimed at achieving the functional recovery of persons affected by neurologic impairment, in subacute and chronic stages, with a potential improvement of the cost/effectiveness ratio. These systems can quantitatively evaluate the effects of rehabilitation treatment and increase the knowledge of motor control and learning mechanisms in humans.

The design of such systems must take into account the ever-increasing knowledge in neurophysiology in order to improve motor function through stimulating, entertaining exercises, and they must be able to engage and motivate the patient.

Several studies have already shown that the use of robotic systems for the rehabilitation of upper and lower limbs can positively contribute to motor recovery in both adult and paediatric patients.

The use of robotic systems for rehabilitation, mechatronic systems for movement analysis and functional assessment, and advanced brain imaging techniques for analysis of the mechanisms of motor recovery for each patient must be integrated in order to define and customize treatment to optimize the hospitalization's period and to husband healthcare resources (Fig. 8).

Furthermore, the development of low-cost robotic systems together with safe, reliable, and robust telecommunications networks can also contribute to the validation of innovative telerehabilitation protocols which may yield great advantages by (i) allowing the rehabilitation process at home or resident care (for the patient), and (ii) reducing the costs associated with hospitalization and rehabilitation at the hospital (for the healthcare system).

Finally, the collaboration between physiatrists, therapists, patients, and engineers, which has already yielded important clinical and scientific results, must be strengthened through research projects and specific programmes at local and national levels, as they are essential for the development of safe and effective technological systems for a patient-oriented robotics programme aimed at improving the quality of life of disabled persons.

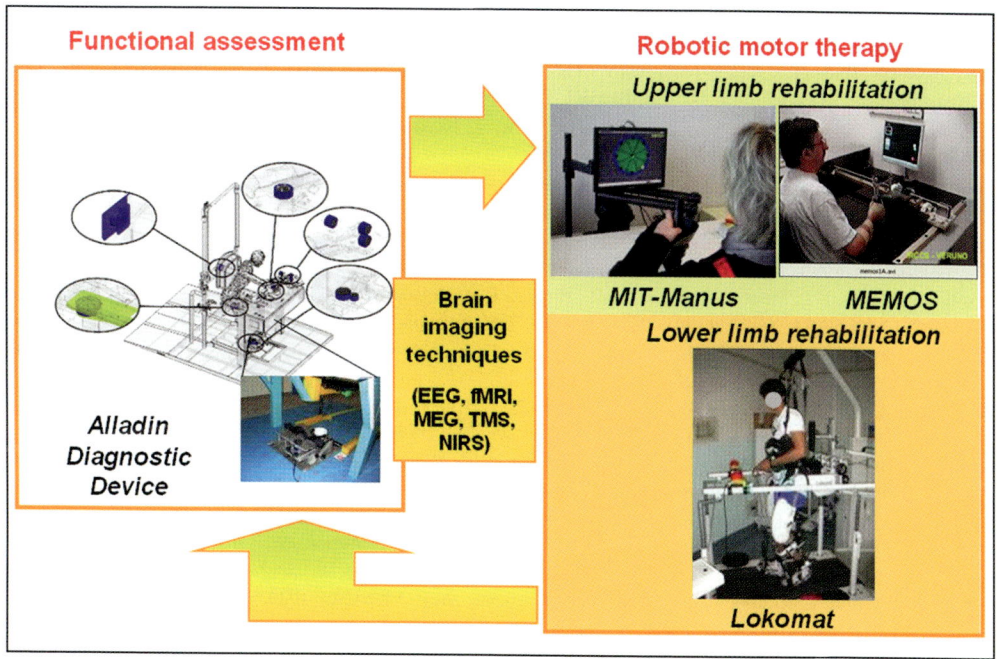

Fig. 8. Robotic and mechatronic systems for rehabilitation: an integrated approach.

**Acknowledgments:** For their help we thank Rehabilitation Centre 'Auxilium Vitae', Volterra, Italy; Rehabilitation Centre 'Auxilium Vitae', Volterra, Italy; Neurorehabilitation Unit, Azienda Ospedaliera Universitaria Pisana, Italy; Fondazione Cassa di Risparmio di Volterra, Italy; Comitato Volterra Ricerche, Italy; Regione Toscana, Italy.

## References

Barbeau, H. & Rossignol, S. (1987): Recovery of locomotion after chronic spinalization in the adult spinal cat. *Brain Res.* **412,** 84–95.

Barbeau, H. & Rossignol, S. (1994): Enhancement of locomotor recovery following spinal cord injury. *Curr. Opin. Neurol.* **7,** 517–524.

Barbeau, H., Ladouceur, M., Norman, K.E. & Pepin, A. (1999): Walking after spinal cord injury: evaluation, treatment, and functional recovery. *Arch. Phys. Med. Rehabil.* **80,** 225–235.

Barbeau, H., Nadeau, S. & Garmeau, C. (2006): Physical determinants, emerging concepts, and training approaches in gait of individuals with spinal cord injury. *J. Neurotrauma* **23,** 571–585.

Borggraefe, I., Kiwull, L., Schaefer, J.S., Koerte, I., Blaschek, A., Meyer-Heim, A. & Heinen, F. (2010): Sustainability of motor performance after robotic-assisted treadmill therapy in children: an open, non-randomized baseline-treatment study. *Eur. J. Phys. Rehabil. Med.* **46,** 125-131.

Borggraefe, I., Meyer-Heim, A., Kumar, A., Schaefer, J.S., Berweck, S. & Heinen, F. (2008): Improved gait parameters after robotic-assisted locomotor treadmill therapy in a 6-year-old child with cerebral palsy. *Mov. Disord.* **23,** 280–283.

Colombo, R., Pisano, F., Micera, S., Mazzone, A., Delconte, C., Carrozza, M.C., et al. (2005): Robotic techniques for upper limb evaluation and rehabilitation of stroke patients. *IEEE Trans. Neural Sys. Rehab. Eng.* **13,** 311–324.

Colombo, R., Pisano, F., Micera, S., Mazzone, A., Delconte, C., Carrozza, M.C., et al. (2008): Assessing mechanisms of recovery during robot-aided neurorehabilitation of the upper limb. *Neurorehabil. Neural Rep.* **22,** 50–63.

Colombo, G., Joerg, M., Schreier, R. & Dietz, V. (2000): Treadmill training of paraplegic patients using a robotic orthosis. *J. Rehabil. Res. Dev.* **37,** 693–700.

Colombo, G., Wirz, M. & Dietz, V. (2001): Driven gait orthosis for improvement of locomotor training in paraplegic patients. *Spinal Cord.* **39,** 252–255.

Dario, P., Guglielmelli, E., Carrozza, M.C., Micera, S., Dipietro, L. & Pisano, F. (2003): Sistemi meccatronici e robotici per la neuroriabilitazione. In: *Bioingegneria della Postura e del Movimento*, Bressanone (Italy). Bologna: Pàtron.

Dietz, V. & Colombo, G. (2004): Recovery from spinal cord injury: underlying mechanisms and efficacy of rehabilitation. *Acta Neurochir. Suppl.* **89,** 95–100.

Donoghue, J.P., Hess, G. & Sanes, J.N. (1996): Motor cortical substrates and mechanisms for learning. In: *Acquisition of Motor Behavior in Vertebrates*, eds. J.R. Bloedel, T.J. Ebner & S.P. Wise, pp. 63–386. Cambridge, MA: MIT Press.

Duncan, P.W., Goldstein, L.B., Matchar, D., Divine, G.W. & Feussner, J. (1992): Measurement of motor recovery after stroke. *Stroke* **23,** 1084–1089.

Edgerton, V.R., Kim, S.L., Ichiyama, R.M., Gerasimenko, Y.P. & Roy, R.R. (2006): Rehabilitative therapies after spinal cord injury. *J. Neurotrauma* **23,** 560–570.

Fasoli, S.E., Krebs, H.I., Stein, J., Frontera, W.R. & Hogan, N. (2003): Effects of robotic therapy on motor impairment and recovery in chronic stroke. *Arch. Phys. Med. Rehabil.* **84,** 477-482.

Fasoli, S.E., Krebs, H.I., Stein, J., Frontera, W.R., Hughes, R. & Hogan, N. (2004): Robotic therapy for chronic motor impairments after stroke: follow-up results. *Arch. Phys. Med. Rehabil.* **85,** 1106-1111.

Fasoli, S.E., Fragala-Pinkham, M., Hughes, R., Hogan, N., Krebs, H.I. & Stein, J. (2008): Upper limb robotic therapy for children with hemiplegia. *Am. J. Rehab.* **87,** 929–936.

Feigin, V.L., Lawes, C.M., Bennett, D.A. & Anderson, C.S. (2003). Stroke epidemiology: a review of population-based studies of incidence, prevalence, and case-fatality in the late 20th century. *Lancet Neurol,* **2,** 43–53.

Ferraro, M., Palazzolo, J.J., Krol, J., Krebs, H.I., Hogan, N. & Volpe, B.T. (2003): Robot aided sensorimotor arm training improves outcome in patients with chronic stroke. *Neurology* **61,** 1604–1607.

Frascarelli, F., Masia, L., Di Rosa, G., Cappa, P., Petrarca, M. Castelli, E. & Krebs, H.I. (2009): The impact of robotic rehabilitation in children with acquired or congenital movement disorders. *Eur. J. Phys. Rehabil. Med.* **45,** 135–141.

Grasso, R., Ivanenko, Y.P., Zago, M., Molinari, M., Scivoletto, G., Castellano, V., et al. (2004): Distributed plasticity of locomotor pattern generators in spinal cord injured patients. *Brain* **127,** 1019–1034.

Harashima, F., Tomizuka, M. & Fukuda, T. (1996): Mechatronics – what is it, why, and how? An editorial. *IEEE/ASME Trans. Mechatron.* **1,** 1–4.

Heart Disease and Stroke Statistics (2009): Update: A Report from the American Heart Association Statistics Committee and Stroke Statistics Subcommittee. Available at: http://circ.ahajournals.org/cgi/reprint/circulationaha.108.191261v1

Hendricks, H.T., Van Limbeek, J., Geurts, A.C. & Zwarts, M.J. (2002): Motor recovery after stroke: a systematic review of the literature. *Arch. Phys. Med. Rehabil.* **83,** 1629–1637.

Hidler, J.M. & Wall, A.E. (2005): Alterations in muscle activation patterns during robotic-assisted walking. *Clin. Biomechan.* **20,** 184–193.

Hidler, J., Nichols, D., Pelliccio, M., Brady, K., Campbell, D.D., Kahn, J.H. & Hornby, T.G. (2009): Multicenter randomized clinical trial evaluating the effectiveness of the Lokomat in subacute stroke. *Neurorehabil. Neural Rep.* **23**, 5–13.

Hogan, N., Krebs, H.I., Sharon, A. & Charnnarong, J. (1995): Interactive Robotic Therapist. U.S. Patent 5, 466, 213.

Hornby, T.G., Campbell, D.D., Kahn, J.H., Demott, T., Moore, J.L. & Roth, H. (2008): Enhanced gait-related improvements after therapist- versus robotic-assisted locomotor training in subjects with chronic stroke: a randomized controlled study. *Stroke* **39**, 1786–1792.

Israel, J.F., Campbell, D.D., Kahn, J.H. & Hornby, T.G. (2006): Metabolic costs and muscle activity patterns during robotic- and therapist-assisted treadmill walking in individuals with incomplete spinal cord injury. *Phys. Ther.* **86**, 1466–1478.

Jezernik, S., Schärer, R., Colombo, G. & Morari, M. (2003): Adaptive robotic rehabilitation of locomotion: a clinical study in spinally injured individuals. *Spinal Cord*, **41**, 657–666.

Koenig, A., Wellner, M., Köneke, S., Meyer-Heim, A., Lünenburger, L. & Riener, R. (2008): Virtual gait training for children with cerebral palsy using the Lokomat gait orthosis. *Stud. Health Technol. Inform.* **132**, 204–209.

Krebs, H.I., Hogan, N., Aisen, M.L. & Volpe, B.T. (1998): Robot-aided neurorehabilitation. *IEEE Trans. Rehab. Eng.* **6**, 75–87.

Krebs, H.I., Volpe, B.T., Aisen, M.L. & Hogan, N. (2000): Increasing productivity and quality of care: robot-aided neuro-rehabilitation. *J. Rehabil. Res. Dev.* **37**, 639–652.

Kwakkel, G., Kollen, B.J. & Krebs, H.I. (2008): Effects of robot-assisted therapy on upper limb recovery after stroke: a systematic review. *Neurorehab. Neural Rep.* **22**, 111–121.

Lum, P.S., Burgar, C.G., Shor, P.C., Majmundar, M. & Van der Loos, M. (2002): Robot-assisted movement training compared with conventional therapy techniques for the rehabilitation of upper-limb motor function after stroke. *Arch. Phys. Med. Rehabil.*, **83**, 952–959.

Lünenburger, L., Colombo, G., Riener, R. & Dietz, V. (2005): Clinical assessments performed during robotic rehabilitation by the gait training robot Lokomat. In: *Proceedings of the 9th International Conference on Rehabilitation Robotics*, pp. 4888–4490. Chicago: Institute of Electrical & Electronics Engineering.

Lünenburger, L., Bolliger, M., Czell, D., Müller, R. & Dietz, V. (2006): Modulation of locomotor activity in complete spinal cord injury. *Exp. Brain Res.* **174**, 638–646.

Meyer-Heim, A., Ammann-Reiffer, C., Schmartz, A., Schäfer, J., Sennhauser, F.H., Heinen, F., et al. (2009): Improvement of walking abilities after robotic-assisted locomotion training in children with cerebral palsy. *Arch. Dis. Child.* **94**, 615–620.

Meyer-Heim, A., Borggraefe, I. Ammann-Reiffer, C., Berweck, S., Sennhauser, F.H., Colombo, G., et al. (2007): Feasibility of robotic-assisted locomotor training in children with central gait impairment. *Dev. Med. Child. Neurol.* **49**, 900–906.

Marini, C., Baldassarre, M., Russo, T., De Santis, F., Sacco, S., Ciancarelli, I. & Carolei, A. (2004): Burden of first-ever ischaemic stroke in the oldest old: evidence from a population-based study. *Neurology* **62**, 77–81.

Mazzoleni, S., Stampacchia, G., Cattin, E., Lefevbre, O., Riggio, C., Troncone, M., et al. (2008): Effects of a robot-mediated locomotor training in healthy and spinal cord injured subjects. In: *Proceedings of the 1st National Conference on Bioengineering*, 245–246, Pisa, Italy. Bologna: Pàtron.

Mazzoleni, S., Toth, A., Munih, M., Van Vaerenbergh, J., Cavallo, G., Dario, P. & Guglielmelli, E. (2009): Whole-body isometric force/torque measurements for functional assessment in neuro-rehabilitation: platform design, development and verification. *J. Neuroeng. Rehab.* **6**, 38.

Mehrholz, J., Platz, T., Kugler, J. & Pohl, M. (2008): Electromechanical and robot-assisted arm training for improving arm function and activities of daily living after stroke. *Cochrane Database of Systematic Reviews* **4**, CD006876.

Micera, S., Mazzoleni, S., Guglielmelli, E. & Dario, P. (2003): Assessment of gait in elderly people using mechatronic devices: preliminary results. *Gait & Posture* **18** (Suppl. 1), S22.

Micera, S., Carpaneto, J., Scoglio, A., Zaccone, F., Freschi, C., Guglielmelli, E. & Dario, P. (2004): On the analysis of knee biomechanics using a wearable biomechatronic device. *Proceedings of the International Conference on Intelligent Robots and Systems* **2**, 1674–1679. Sendai, Japan: Institute of Electrical & Electronic Engineering.

Micera, S., Carrozza, M.C., Guglielmelli, E., Cappiello, G., Zaccone, F., Freschi, C., et al. (2005): A simple robotic system for neurorehabilitation. *Auton. Robots* **19**, 1–11.

Miltner, W.H.R., Bauder, H., Sommer, M., Dettmers, C. & Taub, E. (1999): Effects of constraint-induced movement therapy on chronic stroke patients: a replication. *Stroke* **30**, 586–592.

Murray, C.J.L. & Lopez, A.D. (1997): Global mortality, disability and the contribution of risk factors: global burden of the disease [study]. *Lancet* **349**, 1436–1442.

Nichols-Larsen, D.S., Clark, P.C., Zeringue, A., Greenspan, A. & Blanton, S. (2005): Factors influencing stroke survivors' quality of life during subacute recovery. *Stroke* **36,** 1480–1484.

Petrarca, M., Zanelli, G., Patanè, F., Frascarelli, F., Cappa, P. & Castelli, E. (2009): Reach-to-grasp interjoint coordination for moving object in children with hemiplegia. *J. Rehabil. Med.* **41,** 995–1002.

Posteraro, F., Mazzoleni, S., Aliboni, S., Cesqui, B., Battaglia, A., Dario, P. & Micera, S. (2009): Robot-mediated therapy for paretic upper limb of chronic patients following neurological injury. *J. Rehab. Med.* **41,** 976-980.

Posteraro, F., Mazzoleni, S., Aliboni, S., Cesqui, B., Battaglia, A., Carrozza, M.C., *et al.* (2010): Upper limb spasticity reduction following active training: a robot-mediated study in chronic hemiparetic patients. *J. Rehab. Med.* **42,** 279–281.

Riener, R., Nef, T. & Colombo, G. (2005a): Robot-aided neurorehabilitation of the upper extremities. *Med. Biol. Eng. Comput.* **43,** 2–10.

Riener, R., Lünenburger, L., Jezernik, S., Anderschitz, M. & Colombo, G. (2005b): Patient-cooperative strategies for robot-aided treadmill training: first experimental results. *IEEE Trans. Neural Syst. Rehabil. Eng.* **13,** 380–394.

Riener, R., Lünenburger, L. & Colombo, G. (2006): Human-centered robotics applied to gait training and assessment, *J. Rehab. Res. Dev.* **43,** 679–694.

Schmidt, H., Werner, C., Bernhardt, R., Hesse, S. & Krüger, J. (2007): Gait rehabilitation machines based on programmable footplates. *J. Neuroeng. Rehabil.* **4,** 2.

Scivoletto, G., Ivanenko, Y., Morganti, B, Grasso, R., Zago, M., Lacquaniti, F., *et al.* (2007): Plasticity of spinal centers in spinal cord injury patients: new concepts for gait evaluation and training. *Neurorehabil. Neural Rep.* **21,** 358–365.

Scivoletto, G. & Di Donna, V. (2009): Prediction of walking recovery after spinal cord injury. *Brain Res. Bull.* **78,** 43–51.

SPREAD, Stroke Prevention and Educational Awareness Diffusion (2010): *Ictus cerebrale: linee guida italiane di prevenzione e trattamento*, 6th ed., eds. G.F. Gensini & A. Zaninelli. Milan: Pierrel Research Italy S.p.A. – Catel Division.

Volpe, B.T., Krebs, H.I., Hogan, N., Edelsteinn, L., Diels, C.M. & Aisen, M.L. (1999): Robot training enhanced motor outcome in patients with stroke maintained over 3 years. *Neurology* **53,** 1874–1876.

Volpe, B.T., Krebs, H.I., Hogan, N., Edelstein, L., Diels, C.M. & Aisen, M.L. (2000): A novel approach to stroke rehabilitation: robot aided sensory motor stimulation. *Neurology* **54,** 1938–1944.

Wirz, M., Zemon, D.H., Rupp, R., Scheel, A., Colombo, G., Dietz, V. & Hornby, T.G. (2005): Effectiveness of automated locomotor training in patients with chronic incomplete spinal cord injury: a multicenter trial. *Arch. Phys. Med. Rehabil.* **86,** 672–680.

WHO (World Health Organization): *The atlas of heart disease and stroke*. <http://www.who.int/cardiovascular_diseases/resources/atlas/en/>

Wolf, S.L., Winstein, C.J., Miller, J.P., Taub, E., Uswatte, G., Morris D., *et al.* (2006): Effect of constraint-induced movement therapy on upper extremity function 3 to 9 months after stroke: the EXCITE randomized clinical trial. *JAMA* **296,** 2095–2104.

# Mariani Foundation
# Paediatric Neurology Series

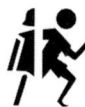

**1: Occipital Seizures and Epilepsies in Children**
Edited by: *F. Andermann, A. Beaumanoir, L. Mira, J. Roger and C.A. Tassinari*
**2: Motor Development in Children**
Edited by: *E. Fedrizzi, G. Avanzini and P. Crenna*
**3: Continuous Spikes and Waves during Slow Sleep – Electrical Status Epilepticus during Slow Sleep**
Edited by: *A. Beaumanoir, M. Bureau, T. Deonna, L. Mira and C.A. Tassinari*
**4: Metabolic Encephalopathies: Therapy and Prognosis**
Edited by: *S. Di Donato, R. Parini and G. Uziel*
**5: Neuromuscular Diseases during Development**
Edited by: *F. Cornelio, G. Lanzi and E. Fedrizzi*
**6: Falls in Epileptic and Non-Epileptic Seizures during Childhood**
Edited by: *A. Beaumanoir, F. Andermann, G. Avanzini and L. Mira*
**7: Abnormal Cortical Development and Epilepsy – From Basic to Clinical Science**
Edited by: *R. Spreafico, G. Avanzini and F. Andermann*
**8: Limbic Seizures in Children**
Edited by: *G. Avanzini, A. Beaumanoir and L. Mira*
**9: Localization of Brain Lesions and Developmental Functions**
Edited by: *D. Riva and A. Benton*
**10: Immune-Mediated Disorders of the Central Nervous System in Children**
Edited by: *L. Angelini, M. Bardare and A. Martini*
**11: Frontal Lobe Seizures and Epilepsies in Children**
Edited by: *A. Beaumanoir, F. Andermann, P. Chauvel, L. Mira and B. Zifkin*
**12: Hereditary Leukoencephalopathies and Demyelinating Neuropathies in Children**
Edited by: *G. Uziel, F. Taroni*
**13: Neurodevelopmental Disorders: Cognitive/Behavioural Phenotypes**
Edited by: *D. Riva, U. Bellugi and M.B. Denckla*
**14: Autistic Spectrum Disorders**
Edited by: *D. Riva and I. Rapin*

**15: Neurocutaneous Syndromes in Children**
Edited by: *P. Curatolo and D. Riva*
**16: Language: Normal and Pathological Development**
Edited by: *D. Riva, I. Rapin and G. Zardini*
**17: Movement Disorders in Children: a Clinical Update, with video recordings**
Edited by: *N. Nardocci and E. Fernandez-Alvarez*
**18: Mental Retardation**
Edited by: *D. Riva, S. Bulgheroni and C. Pantaleoni*
**19: Perinatal Brain Damage: From Pathogenesis to Neuroprotection**
Edited by: *L.A. Ramenghi, P. Evrard and E. Mercuri*
**20: Genetics of Epilepsy and Genetic Epilepsies**
Edited by: *G. Avanzini and J. Noebels*
**21: Neurology of the Infant**
Edited by: *F. Guzzetta*
**22: Brain Lesion Localization and Developmental Functions**
**Basal ganglia – Connecting systems – Cerebellum – Mirror neurons**
Edited by: *D. Riva and C. Njiokiktjien*
**23: Lysosomal Storage Diseases: Early Diagnosis and New Treatments**
Edited by: *R. Parini, G. Andria*

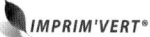 IMPRIM'VERT®

Achevé d'imprimer par Corlet, Imprimeur, S.A.
14110 Condé-sur-Noireau
N° d'Imprimeur : 137716 - Dépôt légal : juillet 2011
*Imprimé en France*